YOUR BODY IN MOTION

What **YOU** Need to Know to Move Better

Karen A. Correia, PT, PhD

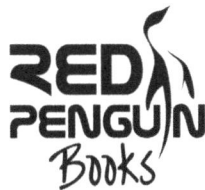

RED PENGUIN
Books

Your Body in Motion: What YOU Need to Know to Move Better

Copyright © 2024 by Karen A. Correia, PT, PhD

Published by Red Penguin Books
Bellerose Village, New York

Library of Congress Control Number: 2023918562

ISBN
Print: 978-1-63777-489-2
Digital: 978-1-63777-490-8

Edited by Janine Logan
Design by KGI Design Group
     Cover Design by Nora Ryder
     Interior Design and Layout by Michelle Fink
Photography, Chapters 10 & 30 by Joseph G. Correia
Photography, Author Headshot and Section Breaks by Len Marks
Photography, Cover by Yuri Arcurs/Shutterstock

This book is meant for educational and demonstration purposes only and is not offering medical advice or medical treatment. The information it contains is not intended to be used for self-diagnosis or to replace medical care. Always consult qualified healthcare providers for advice on medical issues. The information found within does not guarantee better physical movement. Neither the author nor the publisher assumes any liability for any adverse consequences that may result from the information and material presented in this book.

To everyone who wants to move better and/or
help others to move better.

Foreword

When we challenge our movement system to go faster or longer, or when we do new novel activities for work or fun, we may experience muscle and joint aches and pains or less than ideal performance. Whether due to a sport injury, overuse, or misuse of a muscle or a joint, or just general wear and tear on the body, chances are at some point we may have a throbbing knee, stiff back, or some other discomfort that limits our movement. It's not so much the joint, or ligament, or muscle that needs fixing, but it's the way in which we move and use those body parts that might need attention.

This book takes a novel approach to understanding why there may be pain with movement and presents a process for healing that pain. With time and activity, joints deteriorate, tendons are strained, and ligaments stretch unhealthily. The principles about movement taught in this book apply to the body at all stages of development and healing. What you learn here, you may use ten years from now or you may be able to help your children to avoid some of the injuries you experienced because of lack of knowledge. Using the simple analogy of a car, the author teaches about the many body parts involved in movement, and that taking care of these parts may help keep your body, your car, in optimal condition.

Written by Dr. Karen A. Correia, a physical therapist who began her career studying movement as a mechanical engineer and bioengineer, the author draws from her decades of experience working with individuals of all ages from infants to centenarians and a broad range of movement limiting injuries and conditions. She has compiled her extensive clinical and practical knowledge about how the body moves to help you address your movement issues.

The content dives much deeper than the general therapeutic benefits of movement and presents to the reader the why behind exercises. Chapter by chapter, it builds a logical approach to learning about the body and movement and then applies what's learned in a practical way. The book is designed to allow you to teach yourself about movement, injury prevention, and healing. It consists of four parts, starting with how movement is integral to your well-being. This is followed by simple, clear language about the body and how it moves, and progresses to analyzing movement. Once armed with that knowledge, the last part gives tips on how to teach movement. This book is also useful for seasoned physical therapists, physicians, nurses, personal trainers, coaches, martial arts and dance instructors, and others, because of its treatment of movement as a science and therapeutic modality. For all readers, this book provides simple language about movement that may be used to educate patients, clients, family, friends, and colleagues on the movement system.

Treatment of movement issues sometimes focuses on reducing pain rather than identifying and remediating the cause of the pain. Dr. Correia explains that injuries sustained in childhood, long ago but not forgotten by the brain, may be contributing to a pain issue in adulthood. Sometimes, it is the unconscious use of compensating movements that is causing pain and damage. Dr. Correia's book may help you and your movement care team to find the true cause of your pain and movement limitations for lasting improvements in your movement abilities.

*Your Body in Motion: What **YOU** Need to Know to Move Better* stands out from all the other books on this subject because of its emphasis on understanding what movement is, how the body moves, and why. It explains that pain is a message to the brain that something needs to change to allow movement to be safe, efficient, and pain-free. Dr. Correia believes that understanding movement, taking care of the movement system, and making wise movement choices are the foundations to moving well no matter your age or circumstance. Thousands of her patients have benefited from her effective approach and, in fact, many encouraged her to write this book so that others may benefit from her knowledge and methods to move better.

Janine Logan, Editor and Healthcare Writer

Contents

PART 3: Doing

PART 4: Teaching Movement

Introduction

"We shall not cease from exploration and the end of our exploring will be to arrive where we started and know the place for the first time."

– T.S. Eliot[1]

Your Goal: Better Movement With Less Pain

Why should you read this book? Perhaps you have been evaluated by several healthcare providers, attended physical therapy, done your exercises diligently, changed how you move, bought new shoes, and you are still having pain. You want to know why your pain persists. Or, it has become clear to you that if you don't use it, you will lose it. You might be thinking "Is there something else I need to *know*, or is there something I can be *doing* differently to allow me to move better with less pain?" You want to *know* more, so you can *do* better.

You already care for some parts of your body because you want them to last a lifetime. You brush your teeth twice a day to avoid cavities. You clean your glasses before you wear them so you can see clearly without eye strain. You may know how to stretch and strengthen your muscles, but there is much more to *know* and *do* to take care of your movement system.

Learn Tools to Move Better

This book provides you with tools to help you become a better mover. It presents (a) knowledge about the parts of the movement system and how they work together to meet your movement goals, (b) a process for observing and analyzing movement to help identify what may be interfering with good performance or causing pain, and (c) tips on teaching movement.

Learn How the Body Moves

Abusing body parts then replacing them is not the best strategy for taking care of your body. A better plan might be to read the instructions on how your body is supposed to work and learn what you need to know to keep it moving well. *Know* first, *do* second.

This is your opportunity to "Follow the yellow brick road!"[2] to help you reach your destination of the Emerald City of Oz,[3] Kansas, or whatever movement goal you want to achieve. The children's book *The Wonderful Wizard of Oz*[3] is a story about meeting goals. Dorothy wanted to get back to Kansas **(physical)**. The tin man wanted a heart **(emotional)**. The scarecrow wanted a brain **(cognitive)**. The lion wanted courage **(spiritual)**. This book is about knowing more about the physical, emotional, cognitive, and spiritual aspects of movement to help you move better.

Ready, Set, Go

First – Get Ready! Acquire knowledge of individual body parts and how they work together. Second – Get Set! Learn about the physical, emotional, cognitive, and spiritual components of movement. Third – GO! Learn about movement fundamentals and the roles they play in safe, efficient, and pain-free movement.

For you to get the most out of this book, I recommend that you read the book without skipping sections. Like building a house, having a strong, stable, well-aligned foundation – knowledge of the movement system – improves the likelihood that the windows on the second floor – your movements – will open and close smoothly.

Before you *do* anything, like bake a cake or build a table, it is a good idea to *know* your ingredients and your tools and how they are supposed to be used. In terms of your movement system, you may know the names (ingredients) of the parts of your body and perhaps what they do, but you also may benefit from knowing how they work together to perform pain-free movement. Why might you be having pain when you move or what might be interfering with your movement performance? Do you really know which ingredients are underperforming or not "playing well with others?" You may have tried to fix your movement problem by doing the Go! or Do step before the Get Ready! and Get Set! steps. You bought new shoes, added weights to an exercise, or tried a new movement program before you identified the cause of your pain or movement problem. Like any other project, "when all else fails, read the instructions."

How to Use This Book

Read through Parts 1 and 2 to learn about movement before you head into Part 3 to observe movement. Part 4 provides tips for teachers of movement, which essentially is everyone. You may not be a therapist or a coach, but you already have taught yourself how to move. It's probably accurate to say that no parent has instructed their child on how to climb out of a crib or throw toys. How many times have you heard a 2-year-old say, "I did it all by myself."

As poet T.S. Eliot implies, we are always exploring and learning so that we arrive at a point of better understanding. Such is the case with knowing how and why our body moves. It's a good strategy to explore *why* we are having pain or moving poorly before we address how to improve the situation.

While reading this book, you may be awed by how the movement system works and keeps trying to meet your movement goals even if it has to compensate. From experience, you know that compensating too much may put you in a physician's or physical therapist's office. By the time you are a patient, the horse is out of the barn. Something happened and you are having pain, or you have an injury, and you need guidance or treatment. This book focuses on gaining knowledge of how the movement system works and analyzing movement to help keep you on the pickleball court or at work and not in a healthcare provider's office.

When you need to replace a washer in a leaky faucet or cook a chicken using an air fryer, you probably read the instructions first to avoid a catastrophe. Isn't maintaining the health of your body at least as important as a water drip or an overcooked chicken? You may feel you can or want to skip parts of the book (yes, this is your third warning) because either you think you know enough, you don't have the time, or you feel it is too complicated. If you do skip, you may end up having to go back to read the parts you missed because the information in this book builds on previous topics. You need to learn how to walk well before you can skip (pun intended) or run.

Movement is complex because there are many options for getting from point A to point B. What is the best way to get to the grocery store? Option (1) take the safe route and walk on the sidewalk and cross the street at the intersection. Option (2) take the exciting route and walk in between parked cars and cross in the middle of the block. People may experience pain or get injured when they take the wrong route. Knowing the what, the why, and the how of movement may help you choose a better path.

People frequently ask me, "what exercise can I do to make this pain go away?" When I hear this request, I think of the saying, "Give a man a fish and you feed him for a day. Teach a man to fish and you feed him for a lifetime."[4] There are as many exercises and variations as there are fish in the ocean. If I pick one and give it to you, you may be back tomorrow asking me for another exercise because you are having a new pain or you have a new movement goal and yesterday's exercise isn't helping.

This book is intended to teach you what fish (movement components) are available, why you might want to fish in some areas and not others (use one movement option as opposed to another), and some tips for fishing (moving safely) once you are in the right spot. You also will have the opportunity to learn ways to care for your movement system. All this knowledge may be used to improve your ability to fish for whatever type of fish you want, whenever you want, in whatever body of water you choose, and for how long.

This book covers the lifespan from early learning of movement to what happens to the movement system with aging. It also gives some ideas of what may be done to try to slow down the effects of aging. The material is taken from my education and experiences as a physical therapist treating patients of all ages and walks of life with a range of movement problems in a variety of settings. This includes newborns recently released from the neonatal intensive care unit, infants learning how to crawl and walk, preschoolers with developmental delays, teenage athletes, and people of all ages with pain or other issues that interfered with their ability to move well and safely such as construction and computer workers, food preparers, healthcare workers, etc. All people have the same parts, so the concepts of movement apply to everyone. The keys to opening the door to safe, efficient, pain-free movement are to first learn about the 'rules of the road' of the movement system (Part 2) and then about observing and analyzing 'the performance of the car' when doing everyday movements (Part 3).

Do not be tempted to use the excuse that the information presented in this book is "too complicated." Like anything new, you may need to read the information several times before you feel comfortable with it. Learning is a process. You might have struck out your first time at bat, or your first apple pie was a little soggy, but you got better with repetition. Practice makes perfect. I have shared the information in this book with patients many times and have refined the language and examples for better understanding.

The patients I have treated have literally knocked on my door because they wanted to fix their movement problems. The strategies of doing a temporary repair by using pain medication or four to six weeks of exercising was frustrating to them. They wanted to know what to do to take care of themselves to get longer-lasting solutions. Knowledge is power (Part 2).

The subtitle of this book is "What **YOU** need to Know to Move Better" and not "What **YOU** need to Know to Exercise Better." Movement refers to functional activities such as bending, walking, and reaching and skilled activities like hanging a picture, navigating a crowded store, or skiing. Exercise is typically performed to increase flexibility, strength, and muscle and aerobic endurance. Movement programs provide opportunities to practice moving to help you reach your specific movement goals.

What are your movement goals? To walk a greater distance on grass without a cane, to be good enough to make the wrestling or dance team or to be able to stand for a 12-hour shift and play softball afterwards? Perhaps you want to feel more confident when you carry your toddler across an uneven, wet parking lot or you want to bake cookies without needing help? I was motivated to write this book because I was told by many thankful patients "you should write a book." They wanted you to learn about movement so perhaps you might avoid an injury and many hours of physical therapy. So, I present my knowledge and experience to you. The ball is in your court. Set your movement goals and keep reading.

The language used in this book was selected to be understood by everyone including those not in the medical field. The content covers a wide range of topics so you may gain a more complete understanding of the movement system. I use analogies, word pictures, and photos to explain the concepts. When medical terminology is used, the words will be explained to improve clarity. The intention is to provide language that may be used for clear communication between patients or clients, healthcare providers, and movement instructors when solving movement problems.

Movement is life. You move to meet life's goals, share new experiences with friends or, if you are a 2-year-old, you move just because it feels good. So, let's Get Ready! Get Set! and Go!

The Importance of Education

We use knowledge to live safely and happily. A friend of mine might have lived longer if she had been educated on the risk factors of skin cancer and how to recognize an abnormal skin mole. Her plea for us survivors was to educate, educate, educate, on how to take care of our bodies. I hope this book will motivate you to invest in preventative healthcare both for your movement system, as well as the rest of your body. "An ounce of prevention is worth a pound of cure."[5]

My Background in Movement

My perspective on the movement system is based on my experiences as an athlete, physical therapist, educator, and researcher.

1. High school athlete and now participate in fitness activities.

2. Bachelor of Science in Mechanical Engineering where I learned the problem-solving approach that I use for clinical decision-making: define the problem and goals, gather information, apply knowledge of anatomy, kinesiology, and the aging process, develop a solution, carry out appropriate interventions, test the effect of the interventions, and repeat as necessary. I earned a PhD

in Bioengineering where I performed research using computerized motion analysis to study how people walk with canes and crutches.

3. Researched the effects of high-heeled shoes on posture and movement. My desire for a better understanding of *how* the movement system works led me to pursue a degree in Physical Therapy. The combination of my engineering and physical therapy degrees gives me a unique perspective to help people move better.

4. Taught kinesiology, biomechanics, technology in rehabilitation, spinal stabilization training, and resolving hip and back pain by treating the foot and ankle.

5. Physical Therapist since 1991, evaluating and treating people across the life-span who have a variety of orthopedic and neurological diagnoses in outpatient, hospital, and home settings.

6. Completed many hours of continuing education on techniques of physical therapy with special interests in manual therapy, the foot, balance, and understanding pain.

I am excited to present my accumulated knowledge to help you make wise movement decisions. Get Ready! Get Set! Let's Go!

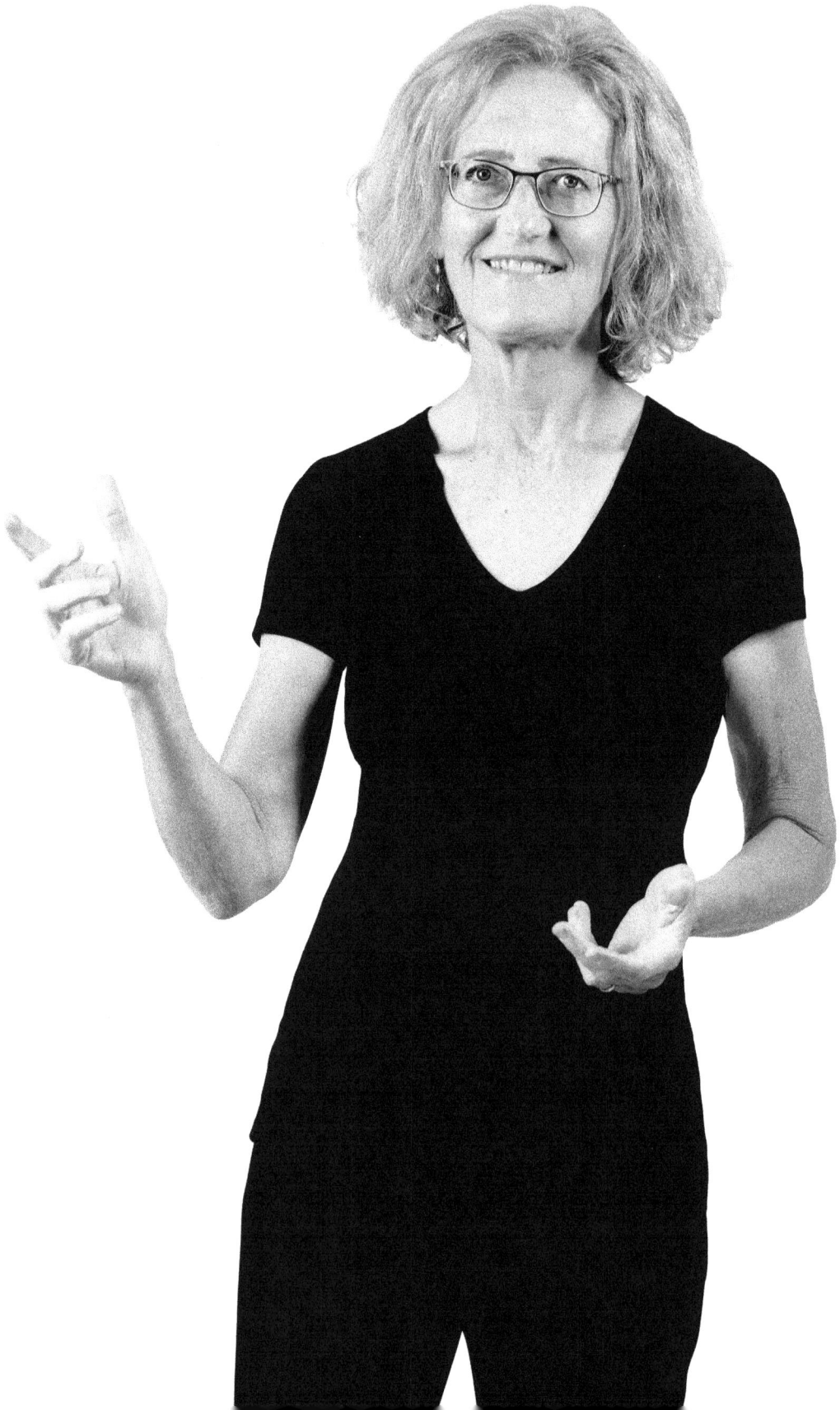

1

It's All About You and Your Well-Being

CHAPTER 1

Moving Better Improves Quality of Life

Feeling happy is an important part of having a good quality of life. You are in the zone of happiness when you express your individuality by doing what you love. You engage in activities like riding a bike or motorcycle, competing in a sport, and/or playing with your grandchildren. All these activities may be more enjoyable when you can move well. With improved movement abilities, you may consider taking on new challenges. You may choose to host a large holiday party, learn a new hobby, or remodel your residence. All these activities require movement.

Do you want to play soccer three times a week, go on more adventurous vacations, or be able to walk your dog without the fear of falling? Perhaps pain, tightness, weakness, or poor endurance are interfering with your enjoyment of life.

Movement plays a big role in your well-being, quality of life, and happiness.[6] Here are some possible physical effects and benefits of physical activity:

Cardiovascular (heart, arteries, veins): increases heart rate and blood pressure to improve circulation. Circulation provides cells and organs with oxygen and nutrition necessary for life and removes waste products of cell metabolism.

Pulmonary (lung): increases depth and rate of breathing to increase oxygen going to cells and organs and carbon dioxide leaving the body.

Gastrointestinal: helps with moving food and gas through the intestines.[7-8]

Lymphatic: assists in flow of lymph, which is important for immune system function.

Neuromusculoskeletal: improves flexibility, strength, endurance, coordination, and balance.

Control of body weight: to help manage diabetes and cardiovascular diseases.

Movement of the head: activates the vestibular system which has a role in muscle tone, balance, and level of alertness.

Cognitive: improves brain function.[9]

In addition to physical health, movement may also enhance emotional or social, cognitive, and spiritual aspects of life. Take another look at the above benefits of movement and see what parts of your life may be impacted by movement: physical, emotional, cognitive, or spiritual.

Movement Is Life

Physically, movement may help to maintain or improve ability to move. **Emotionally**, walking a dog or dancing at a wedding may improve relationship satisfaction and a feeling of well-being. **Cognitively**, challenging the brain to remember sequences by attending a movement class may improve ability to respond to verbal cues in a timely way. **Spiritually**, volunteering and/or doing good deeds for others may be a way of experiencing a more purposeful, fulfilling life. Spirituality may involve giving and contributing, which may be easier when you have physical flexibility, strength, endurance, and coordination. Examples of physical activities that meet spiritual goals are raising a child, cooking for a parent or neighbor, playing music, or teaching a child how to build a birdhouse or sew on a button. The next chapter discusses how meeting your physical, emotional, cognitive, and spiritual goals may cause physiological changes that promote feelings of happiness.

CHAPTER 2

Why Movement Feels Good: Meet Your Neurohormones

Scientists study the brain and the nervous system to try to explain why we are motivated to do certain behaviors and to avoid others.

Finding Happiness in Movement

If you are a parent, a teacher, or a supervisor you probably would like to have children who behave politely and respectfully, students who study, and employees who are productive. These behaviors may involve, you guessed it, movement. When movements are accomplished successfully, the brain has a process for releasing chemicals that may lead to feelings of fulfillment and happiness (discussed below).

Sometimes movement may lead to injury, fatigue, and more pain – not a happy scenario. An example of this might be someone who has not maintained the flexibility and strength of their legs and is having knee pain and difficulty keeping up with their three-year-old grandchild.

The take-home message: keeping your body moving well may help improve your level of happiness.

While the workings of the brain and nervous system are complex, scientists are generally in agreement with this simplified statement: the body has the ability to release specific chemicals that contribute to you feeling good or happy.[6,10-11] A question you might ask is "How do we get the body to release these chemicals and at the same time carry out our responsibilities as a student, worker, or caregiver?"

The Neuroscience of Happiness

Here is a brief neuroscience lecture on happiness. The nervous system plays a role in all body functions including heart rate, digestion, thoughts, memory, feelings, hormone regulation, sensation of hunger, and senses of sight, touch, and more. The body has billions of nerve cells that interconnect to send messages to and from the brain to carry out all these functions. Neurotransmitters and neurohormones are some of the chemicals that either pass on or prevent messages from going to other nerves nearby or remotely. Thoughts may also trigger the release of neurohormones and the hormone cortisol. These chemicals may affect many parts of the body including the functioning of the autonomic nervous system, which controls heart rate, blood pressure, breathing rate, immune system function, and digestion. In sum, the neurohormones and the cortisol hormone that are released in your body may affect how you feel physically.

While being happy is unique to the individual, most would agree that 'feeling good' is a happy state.

The 'Feel-Good' Neurohormones[6,10-11]

It is interesting that the body has neurohormones that can affect the quality of life that was discussed in the previous chapter: physical (dopamine), emotional (oxytocin), and cognitive/spiritual (serotonin).

Dopamine. This neurohormone is released when you experience or anticipate getting your needs met, a reward, or something pleasant. Examples might be getting credit for doing a good job, eating a piece of peach pie and ice cream, or looking forward to an island vacation.

Oxytocin. This neurohormone is released with you feel accepted socially and you feel safe. Perhaps you wear clothes that your girlfriend or boyfriend likes, or you may try playing pickleball because everyone else is doing it.

Serotonin. This neurohormone is released when you feel the respect of others or pride in yourself. You are the first one in your group to install a new phone app or you are strong enough to carry your luggage up the stairs.

Three themes of the above authors are 1) dopamine, oxytocin, and serotonin are linked to our survival, 2) exercise and movement may stimulate a neurohormone release leading to feeling good and happy, and 3) we are motivated to do certain behaviors because we seek the reward of the good feeling that we get from a neurohormone release.

The Stress Hormone Cortisol

Cortisol is typically released in stressful situations. Cortisol may be good or bad. Cortisol is good when it is released in response to a 'fight or flight' situation such as when there is pain or the potential for bodily harm. Heart rate, blood pressure and blood sugar levels increase. Blood vessels increase or decrease in size which changes blood flow to improve muscle function at the expense of maintenance functions of the body such as digesting food.

Cortisol may also be released when there is an emotional stress such as anxiety before a test or speaking in public. In these situations, cortisol activates the sympathetic nervous system to prepare the body to 'fight or flee' from stress even though there is no intention of fighting or fleeing. At other times, the body 'rests and digests,' the roles of the parasympathetic nervous system which promotes body maintenance and an environment for healing. Frequent or extended cortisol releases and extended time spent in the sympathetic mode may lead to disease states such as hypertension, diabetes, depression, weight gain, and sleeping disorders.

In sum, cortisol is beneficial when you need to survive by fighting or fleeing but may not be so good for your cardiovascular or digestive systems if it is released too frequently.

Getting the Benefits of Neurohormones

Can movement promote the release of the feel-good neurohormones in your body? Here are some possibilities:

"When I can do the whole 45 minutes of the movement class, I am going to buy those new shoes." Dopamine: anticipation of a reward.

"Since I improved my endurance on the bicycle, I was able to keep up with my friends on the Saturday morning bike ride." Oxytocin released: accepted by the group.

"When I started, I could only lift 5 pounds. Now I can hold 10 pounds while walking up and down two flights of stairs." Serotonin released: feelings of accomplishment and pride.

Is It Really Mind Over Matter?

It very well may be mind over matter. Try a behavior that is linked to a release of dopamine, oxytocin, or serotonin and see if you get the good feeling from a neuro-hormone release. It is important that you set goals, engage in behaviors, and strive for rewards that meet *your* needs. This may require some self-assessment to identify what is important to you. If the goal is a physical activity, you may benefit from someone helping you assess your abilities to establish achievable goals. More on this very important topic of self-assessment and goal setting in Chapter 7.

CHAPTER 3

The Difference Between Exercise and Movement

Exercise and movement are similar, but they usually have different purposes. In general, the goal of exercise is to help you move better. Goals of movement tend to be purposeful like walking downstairs to do the laundry so you can have clean clothes for play or work, or engaging in a round of golf because you enjoy the sport and being with your friends. Exercise tends to be repetitive while movement typically incorporates a variety of postures and interactions with the surrounding environment.

Exercise

There are many reasons why you may like to exercise. It makes you feel good. You want to get stronger to be fit for your upcoming vacation in the mountains. Or you want to look good when you are with family and friends (serotonin, dopamine, and oxytocin jolts).

There are many reasons why you may *not* like to exercise. You may think it is a lot of sweaty work without a purpose. You may feel that it needs to be done to a certain standard and you don't want to be judged by how you perform. Or maybe you don't see how exercise helps you meet your movement goals or relieve your pain.

Typically, exercise involves activities that are done repetitively in a controlled environment. Exercise activities are usually done with the body moving in one direction like walking on a treadmill or lifting weights and the level of difficulty is increased by increasing time, weights or repetitions.

Generally, exercises are performed to improve posture, strength, balance, flexibility, and endurance.[12] Cardiovascular exercise like bicycling, rowing, or jogging is performed to improve cardiovascular endurance.

Movement

Movement typically refers to activities where the body uses many joints and muscles to achieve a goal such as walking across a street to get to the hair salon or barber shop or reaching to get a plate off a shelf. Some movements in life are predictable like getting into or out of a car or reaching down to pick up a shoe. Exercise may be helpful for maintaining the abilities to do these movements. Movements may be performed in response to an unpredictable, new, or changing environment. In addition to flexibility, strength, and endurance, a movement may require weight shifting, coordination, and balance. These latter abilities may be improved by participating in movement programs.

Typically, movement programs involve many body parts and a variety of postures and movements – reaching with the feet next to each other, reaching while taking one step forward, etc. Examples of movement programs include yoga, Tai Chi, martial arts, fitness and dance and balance classes, etc. Movement programs may incorporate postures and movements that are done every day: bending to get something off a low shelf, lunging to keep a toddler out of mischief, or reaching to hang up a jacket or replace a shower curtain. Movement programs may incorporate a range of speeds that correspond to how activities are performed throughout the day.

A goal of both exercise and movement programs is to engage in activities that increase your ability to move safely and efficiently.

The following is an example of two strategies that may be used to meet a movement goal. Your goal is to be able to get up from a chair that does not have armrests. Being able to get up from a chair without armrests may be an important goal for you because it increases your independence so you can go out to eat with your friends or family (oxytocin jolt) and be able to use the restroom without assistance.

Perhaps you are unable to meet your goal of getting up from a chair without armrests because your legs are weak. Or perhaps you do not have enough flexibility or balance.

You may not know what is limiting you, but you might assume that you are weak, and you start a general strengthening exercise program. A strategy that may be more successful for you is to have someone identify the deficits that are limiting the movement, then engage in specific flexibility, strengthening, and/or balance programs that address those limitations. By engaging in the first strategy, you may get stronger, but that may not help you get up from a chair without armrests if balance was your limiting factor. I call this first strategy 'frosting a stale cake.' You can frost your cake with chocolate icing (make some muscles stronger), but for the whole cake to taste good (for you to get up from the chair without armrests easily) you may be more successful if you identify and overcome the *cause* of the problem (why the cake is stale).

Strive for Movement-Based Goals

Going back to the discussion on happiness, successful movements that help you to accomplish your work, play, and activities of daily living goals may provide neurohormone releases. Patients may not be compliant with a physician's or therapist's prescription for exercise because they may not understand how exercise is going to help them move better. Healthcare providers and movement instructors may be able to help their patients and clients get better physically and have improved compliance if they know their patients' physical, emotional, cognitive, and spiritual goals. Then the patient/client and provider may collaborate to develop exercise and/or movement programs to improve the physical abilities that are needed to help the patient/client reach their movement goals. Healthcare providers know that the physical body declines with age even in the absence of disease, but patients may not be aware of this. The phrase "golden years are not so golden" hopefully will not be true for you. Patients, clients, healthcare providers, and movements instructors working together is a good strategy to optimize movement abilities before and during the golden years.

CHAPTER 4

Motivated to Move

Fear is a great motivator for change. You have heard the words "use it or lose it." You may be experiencing this situation now. Simply put, due to the aging process, you may want to consider using/moving your body, or you may be faced with losing your ability to move it.

It is normal for physical abilities to decline with age (Chapter 22). By doing your routine, daily movements, you may be merely maintaining your movement abilities. If there is a day when you need to walk further or faster or go up a flight of stairs carrying a 15-pound bag of groceries, you may not be able to do so.

The 'Movement Ability Bank'

You may be saving money in a bank account (or elsewhere) for a rainy day when you need it for an unexpected expense. Have you considered using the same wisdom with your body? Increase your movement abilities in your 'movement ability bank' so they are available when you need them to perform a challenging movement. If you are around 25 or 30 years old, your 'rainy day' may be just a light drizzle which doesn't interfere with your movements. At age 60, your 'rainy day' may require an umbrella. To be clear, with passing time, you may lose some of your movement abilities – flexibility, strength, speed of movement, endurance – if you are not challenging them. You already may be concerned about a decline in your movement abilities. Don't let this feeling overwhelm you. Give yourself a serotonin jolt by engaging in appropriate exercise and movement programs to help maintain and improve your abilities.

Chapter 2 explained how the nervous system and its neurohormones might play a role in motivation and behaviors. Movement may cause a release of dopamine, oxytocin, and serotonin 'feel-good' neurohormones and be a win-win-win-win for your physical, emotional, cognitive, and spiritual states. Develop short- and long-term goals that incorporate movement. Like money in the bank, having more physical abilities provides you with more options. When you need to respond to a challenging task such as a loss of balance, you want to be prepared to be able to avoid a fall with its potentially devastating consequences.

The Neurohormone – Movement Cycle

In sum, besides the possible physical benefits, movement may also improve your well-being by helping you to meet emotional, cognitive, and spiritual goals. Your neurohormones may help you to feel good when you move which may motivate you to move more. Move – feel good when you move – improve your ability to move – move more. Awesome!

Let's review:

Movement may allow you to keep working or playing longer (dopamine).

Moving better may help you to be able to keep up with peers physically (oxytocin).

When you move, you may be a role model for the next generation to improve their movement habits and long term well-being (oxytocin).

Movement may help you to feel more capable and respected by peers (serotonin).

Movement may help you to feel good physically and may relieve depression (dopamine, serotonin).[6]

Movement may help to slow down a decline in physical function and maintain independent living with increasing age (serotonin).

Not Moving? Why Not?

You may be someone who has some 'good' reasons for not engaging in a movement program. As a physical therapist, I have heard many of them. I am going to list some for you so you may become aware of why you might be avoiding movement.

A legitimate excuse for not wanting to move more is because you have pain when you do move. If you are in this situation, it might be a good idea to get professional guidance to help identify the cause of the pain. By the way, science has demonstrated that movement may block the sensation of pain, so movement is sometimes recommended for pain relief.[13]

I don't want to move more because of **physical** barriers:

1. I would have to wear clothes that I don't have or am not comfortable in.
2. I am too busy, or it would take too long.
3. I don't have the energy.
4. It would cost too much.
5. I don't have the right equipment.

I don't want to move more because of **emotional** barriers:

1. I am afraid of change.
2. I am afraid of failing.
3. I am depressed and/or anxious.
4. Moving is not fun (may mean that the person is unhappy and is not focusing on how to achieve happiness).
5. I am afraid of not liking the changes in me that may happen.
6. I am afraid of starting something I may not be able to finish.
7. I am afraid of not being able to go back to my old self if I stop.
8. I am afraid I won't be able to maintain my new self.
9. People may not like the new me.
10. I don't trust anyone, so I am not going to ask anyone to help me learn how to move.
11. I may lose a relationship if I become more physically active.

I don't want to move more because of **cognitive** barriers:

1. I don't think it's important.
2. I don't think it can really help me.
3. I don't have any reason to move.
4. I don't think it's physically possible for me to move more.
5. I don't know how.
6. I am too old, or too young, or too overweight, or too underweight.

I don't want to move more because of **spiritual** barriers:

1. I am lazy (may mean I have not found a purpose in life that I want to put effort into).
2. If I maintain my current physical condition, I have an excuse to not cook, go to work, or engage in social situations.
3. I don't need to improve my physical abilities because I can get other people to do physical tasks for me.
4. I want to keep the attention I get when I complain about my physical situation.
5. I am comfortable keeping things the way things are. I can put up with the pain or loss of function.
6. I feel I am not worthy of having a higher level of function.
7. I believe I cannot achieve what I want physically.
8. I believe I am not capable of going through the process (physically, emotionally, cognitively, or spiritually).
9. I don't feel I am responsible for having a role in taking care of myself.

Another barrier to change might be the people you associate with. Are you surrounded by people that support you? Or do people talk you into engaging in tasks that are not a priority for you? Perhaps they discourage you from walking up the stairs because they want to take the elevator. Or maybe they encourage you to hire a house cleaner because they don't like to vacuum even though you see it as good exercise. Consider surrounding yourself with people that encourage you rather than those who distract you or limit you to old behaviors.

If you don't find yourself on the above list, there is one more situation that might be interfering with your choosing to engage in a movement program or any type of change in your life. You may be stuck in the grieving process due to a loss. I extend to you my sympathies for your loss. You may benefit from going through the process of grieving – denial, anger, bargaining, depression, and acceptance.[14] Reaching acceptance frees you up to move on and create good.

The stages of grief for movement may look something like this:

Denial: I really don't have movement deficits. My problem will go away. I am just getting old. What I am experiencing is normal. The numbness in my toes is not such a big deal. The doctor is wrong. My rotator cuff doesn't feel like it's torn even though they tell me it is.

Anger: I am mad that these movement deficits are part of my life and interfering with my goals/fun/happiness. Why me? I didn't do anything wrong.

Bargaining: If I were 30 pounds lighter or I could move without getting short of breath or if I could get good results by adding10 minutes of movement twice a week, then I would participate. I want everything to be better when I buy new shoes or take a pill. If I give it enough time, everything should get better.

Depression: I haven't been moving in so long I don't think anything I do will help me. This is not working out like I expected even after all the changes I made. This is really messing up my life. What am I supposed to do? I can't do what I want to do without pain. I am unhappy and I have lost hope.

Acceptance: I will do the best I can with my torn rotator cuff. Yes, I have a problem. I need to modify my activities to be safe. I don't move enough. If I keep on like this, I won't be able to go on a trip to visit my relatives, go to a pottery class, and/or continue working or volunteering. I have decided to put some time and effort into making movement a part of my life. I think it's time to pursue outside help.

CHAPTER 5

Change or Be Chained

Definition of Change: Adapt. Modify. Revise. Improve.

Definition of Chain: Restrain. Confine.

As you get older, your body changes. Think of your body as something that has value, say $1000. If you do nothing, because of inflation, as time passes the buying power of $1000 is maybe $800. You will get less product or service for your money as time goes on. Your body is the same. If you do nothing, it is normal for your ability to move to lessen over time.

Clearly, to keep your buying power with money or your movement power with your body you need to make modifications, revisions, improvements, adaptations, or investments. Your other option is to be chained, restrained, and confined. Your choice: improve and adapt or be limited in your movement options.

"The only thing we have to fear is fear itself."[15] Fear of change. Fear of the unknown. Make the unknown known. This book provides you with an opportunity to learn more about how your body works and a process to improve your ability to move safely, efficiently, and perhaps with less pain. You may benefit from professional guidance to help you achieve your movement goals. Using their knowledge and experience, health-care providers may be able to provide you with insights on what your health or abilities may be 5, 10, or 15 years from now, if you do not change your current lifestyle and habits. You may choose to make a change now and potentially avoid future problems or you may choose not to change and face the potentially negative consequences. Using a car analogy, when you see the sign 'road closed ahead,' you may decide to proceed on the same road with the possibility that the sign is incorrect or you may turn around and find another road to get you to your destination.

The take-home message is: If you are hesitant to make lifestyle changes to maintain or improve your health, at least get informed on what the consequences of your inaction might be. Ask your healthcare provider what might happen if you don't follow their recommendations. They are not trying to make you fearful. They are trying to communicate urgency, which is an important step in the process of change (see Chapter 6).

If you are a healthcare provider or movement instructor, how might you be rewarded when you help your patients or clients to make lifestyle changes? When explaining health issues and making recommendations, healthcare providers and movement instructors may be rewarded with dopamine (anticipation of a reward that you will feel or move better), serotonin (increased pride that they are competent at providing good care), and oxytocin (feeling a positive connection with you because you engaged them in your process of solving your movement problems).

What Are Your Beliefs?

When I asked people about what they thought was important when they wanted to make a change, some common themes emerged:

1. Change may make you feel uncomfortable until you get used to it.
2. Every day do one thing to move forward on your path to reach your goals.
3. Plan and engage in situations where you may make a mistake. Learning what *not* to do is sometimes more important than learning what to do. When it comes to movement, learning your limitations might help you avoid an injury.
4. Whatever you are doing, make sure you are having fun which is essentially the same as feeling happy.

When you act on the above beliefs, you may be rewarded with neurohormone jolts:

1. Pride from being able to adapt without feeling threatened (serotonin)
2. Anticipation of meeting your goal (dopamine)
3. Pride from learning (serotonin)

4. In any activity that you choose (because fun and happiness are different for different people), you may get a neurohormone reward: getting a need met (dopamine), feeling more socially connected (oxytocin), or feeling respected by others or proud of yourself (serotonin).

Embrace Change

The underlying theme in the above beliefs is change. Change may be physical, emotional, cognitive, and/or and spiritual. Get comfortable with change. Do something each day to change yourself. Today you are reading this book to increase your knowledge of movement. You are investing in yourself. Serotonin jolt for you!

Change or be chained. To maintain or improve your movement abilities, you may engage in an exercise or a movement program, to 'change' your balance, flexibility, etc. or you may choose to do nothing and 'be chained' with the consequences of decreased mobility. Exercise or movement programs do take time and sometimes money to reap the reward. As a physical therapist, I have encountered older adults living in the "golden years" who have time and money, but their physical limitations were preventing them from enjoying vacations and other activities. You choose. Don't allow fear of the unknown, or any of those excuses mentioned in Chapter 4, choose for you.

CHAPTER 6

How-To's of Change

You might be thinking that you can skip this chapter because your life has been nothing but change. You know all you need to know about change. Perhaps there may be something else you can learn about the process of change. Or maybe you will discover a barrier that is interfering with your ability to change.

There are many ways to go about creating change. The process listed below is a possible strategy for changing your movements. Each step has the potential for a neurohormone release.

1. **Create a movement goal**

    Be able to walk 6,000 steps 3 days a week (serotonin). Get in shape for a 50-mile bike ride with a friend in 2 months (serotonin and oxytocin). Be able to perform sit to stand from a chair 6 times in 30 seconds (serotonin). Have enough muscle endurance to do 4 hours of overtime twice a week (serotonin and dopamine).

2. **Create a timeline for your goals and make the goal a priority for you**

    I want to run a 10K race in 4 months and be able to finish in a good time (serotonin). I want to be able to play soccer with my friends next season (oxytocin). I need to learn how to move without pain as soon as possible so I can stop taking pain medication that causes an upset stomach (dopamine). Everyone thinks I'm a weakling. I want to feel stronger (serotonin). I almost fell. I need to do something to decrease my risk of falling (dopamine).

3. **Find someone who supports you**

    Find someone to share your accomplishments with (oxytocin).

4. **Find the barriers to meeting your goal and get rid of them**

   See Chapter 4 for barriers. Become proud of yourself by overcoming barriers (serotonin).

5. **Give yourself frequent rewards**

   Rewards are like gifts to yourself such as words of encouragement, time, things (dopamine), or the feel-good rewards of the releases of dopamine, oxytocin, or serotonin.

6. **Realize the movement goals may keep changing**

   To keep getting the hormone release, you may need to make the reward higher or more stimulating as time goes on (dopamine), increase the quality of the social interaction (oxytocin), or make new goals that make you feel accomplished when you meet them (serotonin). Be able to walk 8,000 steps 3 days a week. Bike 75 miles with a bike club. Be able to perform sit to stand from a chair 8 times in 30 seconds. Have enough muscle endurance to do 4 hours of overtime 3 times a week.

7. **Make the exercise or movement program a part of your life**

   The exercise or movement activities should become part of your routine like brushing your teeth such that you would miss them if you didn't do them. A routine might be to do 30 minutes of yoga 3 times per week, jog 20 minutes every other day, perform resistance training 15 minutes every day alternating upper and lower body exercises, or bike for an hour after work every Tuesday and Thursday (serotonin).

8. **Plan how to implement the change**

   Make the activity a priority. Plan the time, duration, and location of the activity, clothing and equipment, who you are going to do it with, how much energy you want to put into the activity, how fast you want to progress, and how often you want to change your goals. You may be able to add to your neurohormones releases by adding variety – different music, new clothes/footwear, attend a class with a different teacher, or try another path for walking or jogging (dopamine, oxytocin, serotonin).

9. **Self-assess**

    Assess if you are meeting your goals. Modify the exercise or movement program to get the neurohormone you want. You may want to start walking with a neighbor to increase oxytocin or start moving faster or longer or with more resistance to increase serotonin or add another day to your weekly program to get stronger or lose weight faster to get dopamine. It's called **self**-assessment because it's all about **you** and **your well-being** (and your feel-good neurohormones)!

CHAPTER 7

Making Movement Goals

Why is making movement goals a good idea? Goals help to keep you focused and motivated, and you can reward yourself when you meet them.

Goals should be specific, measurable, have a time frame, and be achievable. "I will walk 2 miles outdoors 3 days per week without pain starting June 15" is a good goal. "I will walk more" is not measurable nor does it have a time frame. If you just had knee surgery, you may need to modify the above goal to be less challenging so that there is more likelihood for success: "I will walk 1/2 mile, 3 days per week and increase one day each week until I reach 5 days per week." You may need guidance from a professional to assess your abilities to help you set an achievable goal.

Think about goals that may meet more than one of your needs - physical, emotional, cognitive, and spiritual. Younger people may tend to have goals that address physical and cognitive abilities since their bodies and minds have great potential for improvement. On the other hand, with age there may be lower physical and cognitive abilities, but higher levels of functioning emotionally and spiritually, so goals may relate to meeting needs in these areas.

A younger person's goals may be: "I want to increase my running speed to be able to win my age group for the 5K race, be a master plumber, host a birthday party for 15 toddlers, or canoe across the lake."

An older person with less physical endurance may choose one activity and adapt the situation to get dopamine, oxytocin, and serotonin jolts as well as get their physical, emotional, cognitive, and spiritual needs met. For example, "I will increase my shoulder flexibility and strength so my grandson will want to be my partner when we play cornhole and I will keep score. I want to be an example to him on how to be disciplined about taking care of yourself." By performing one activity, the older person may be able to get releases of dopamine, oxytocin, and serotonin and meet physical, emotional, cognitive, and spiritual goals.

Table 1 shows how movement goals may vary across the lifespan. Physical and cognitive abilities start low and typically improve then decline with age. Emotional abilities may increase with age and may improve or decline with further aging. Spiritual abilities have the potential to keep improving with age depending on the person. Listed are possible movement options. As with any change in your physical movements, seek medical advice before engaging in any of the activities listed in Table 1.

Table 1: Movement Goals Across the Lifespan

Age	Goals
0-10	Learn and practice postures with good techniques when using the phone, computer, and other electronic devices. This goal should be continued through your life. Have fun when engaging in movement activities.
11-20	Challenge physical abilities and gain respect of others or pride in yourself from movement. Increase exposure to a variety of sports, recreational activities, hobbies, and movement experiences.
21-30	Integrate movement into work and social activities. Engage in hobbies and recreational habits that provide opportunities to develop skills to help you stay motivated.
31-40	Integrate movement into daily activities: working, caring for a family, home, or travel.
41-50	Modify or engage in new movements to increase the variety of your movement memories (Chapter 17).
51-60	Include movement in social, travel, and recreational activities.
61-70	In movement activities, consider physical changes that may limit safe participation. Develop movement habits to maintain flexibility, strength, endurance, coordination, balance, and speed of movement.
71-80	Use assistive devices as needed for safety and to maintain flexibility and movement endurance. Consider performing functional activities such as getting up from the floor, stair climbing, and sit to stand without using hands to help maintain independence.
81-110	Find reasons to move: walk instead of drive to the convenience store to get a cup of coffee. Keep up with the movement habits you established during your 60's and 70's.

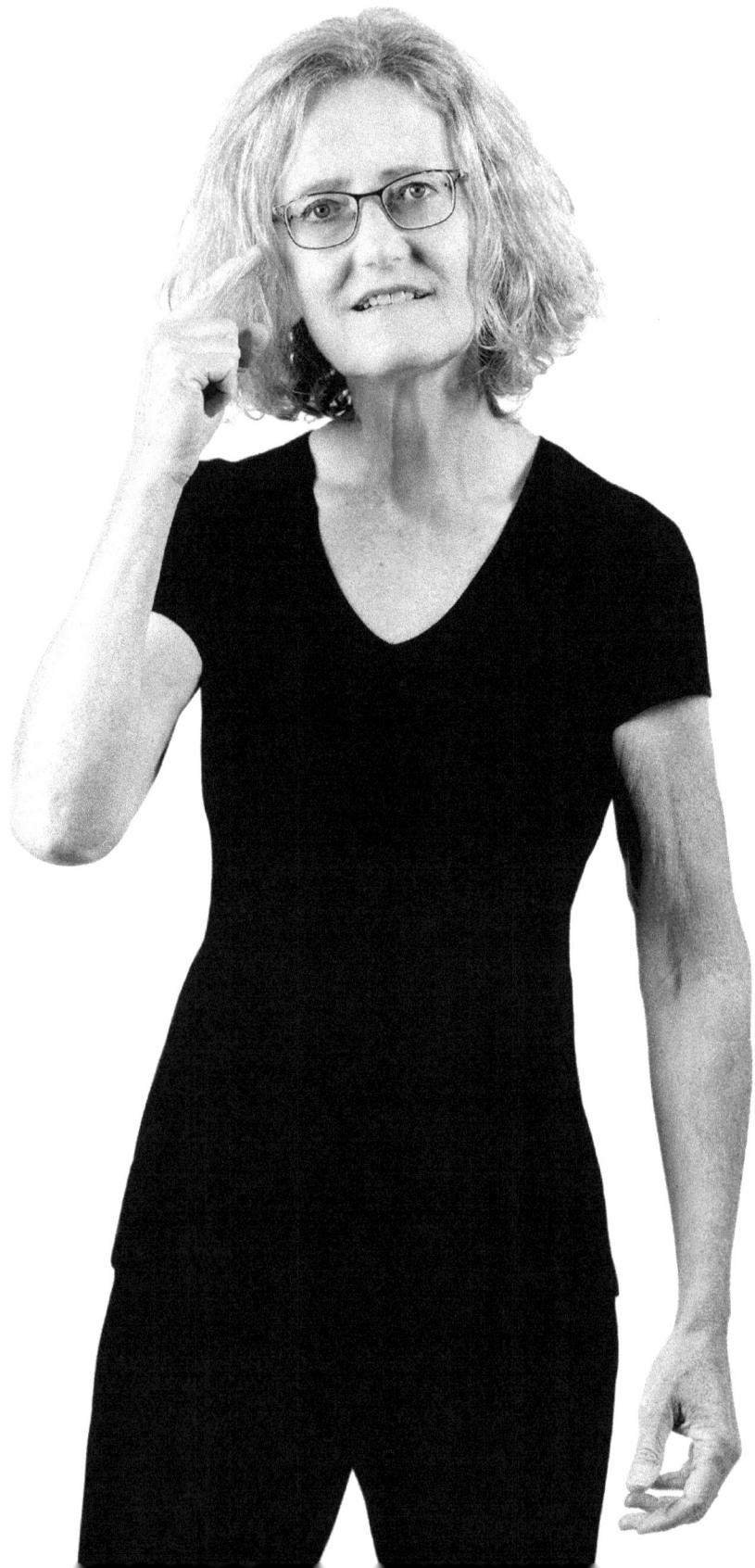

2
Knowing

"Knowledge is Power."

– Francis Bacon[16]

CHAPTER 8

What You Need to Know

As a physical therapist, I am often asked, "What exercise can I do to get rid of the pain in my … (fill in the blank)?" My first thought is, "I wonder if this person asks their mechanic to fix their car without doing diagnostic testing first?" On the positive side, their request does tell me that they have done some self-assessment and that they are aware they have a problem. They also know that what they have done so far hasn't worked. However, they have made a leap by deciding that an exercise to improve flexibility or strength is the solution to making their pain go away. Pain may come from many sources, but tightness or weakness merely describes the state of a muscle and may not be the *cause* of the pain. A mechanic probably would not advise you to use a fuel additive to improve your car's acceleration before they checked the fuel lines, filter, and fuel pump. It might be more appropriate to ask, 'Why do I have pain here when I do this?' A next step might be to evaluate the muscles, tendons, ligaments, and joints that are involved in the movement and palpate to identify structures that may be painful and/or not functioning well. To get a solution for a movement issue that is lasting, just like a car, you may benefit by taking into account *all* the parts that are related to the movement problem. You might be annoyed if you had to go back to the mechanic every six months to 'fix' the same problem. Trying exercise after exercise or increasing rest times to relieve pain without finding the *cause* of the pain may be a frustrating strategy that at best may offer only temporary relief.

This book provides knowledge of the parts of the body, their roles in movement, and how the body may be used efficiently to help improve performance and/or lower the risk of injury. With more knowledge about the movement system, you may be better able to collaborate with your healthcare providers and movement instructors to help you reduce pain and improve function. Treat the *cause*, not the symptom. Success is where opportunity meets preparation. Your opportunity to learn is now. Take a minute and prepare yourself physically, emotionally, cognitively, and spiritually to expand your knowledge on how your amazing body works to be able to provide you with decades of safe, efficient, and pain-free movements.

What Do You Currently Know?

You know you have a movement problem because you are having pain, or your performance is not what you want it to be. You know you want to move better both now and in the future.

You know that what you have tried so far hasn't worked to your satisfaction. You may be thinking you may need to know more about the movement system to help you fix your problem.

If you are a healthcare provider, coach, caregiver, personal trainer, etc., you know how important it is for your patients and clients to move well. You think there might be something more to learn about the movement system that may help you provide better care for your patients and clients.

My goal is for you to be able to help yourself and others with movement challenges. Patients sometimes report to me that they have shared their new knowledge of the movement system, and they see that their children, spouses, and parents are moving better.

What Do You Need to Learn?

With any new project, seeing the 'big picture' helps to organize the pieces. It is easier and quicker to build a jigsaw puzzle when you can look at the picture on the box and see how the objects and colors are related. By knowing the goal, you may lower or eliminate a fear of the unknown. The 'big picture' for movement is illustrated in the Knowing / Doing graphic.

In situations where you want to do something like make an omelet or assemble a piece of furniture, you usually have a mindset. "That looks easy." Or, "That might be too difficult for me." Or, "That looks simple." Or, "That seems complicated." The Knowing / Doing graphic shows the combinations of easy-difficult and simple-complex that may be your mindset. A task in the left upper quadrant might be complex, but it can be performed easily. That is, there are a lot of parts and connections making it *complex*, but each connection is *easy* to assemble. A task in the lower right quadrant might be *simple* – connect part A to part B – but it is very *difficult* to do because it needs to be done with fine tools using a microscope.

Figure 1: Knowing / Doing

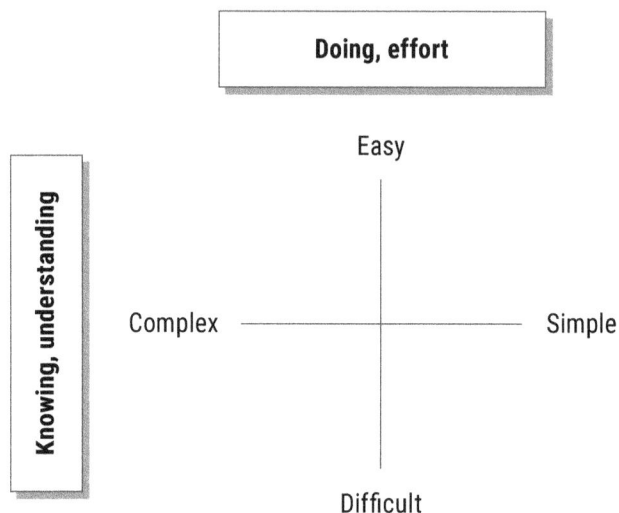

Doing, effort

Easy

Knowing, understanding

Complex ——————————+—————————— Simple

Difficult

Where you stand on the Know / Doing graphic is based on your knowledge, your experience, and your physical abilities. Depending on how much you know about cooking and how your stove works and your hand dexterity, making an omelet may be complex or simple or difficult or easy. In assembling furniture, your knowledge of wood and screws and your ability to use a screwdriver determines whether you think the project is complex or simple or difficult or easy. Basically, with more *knowledge* tasks become simpler, and with more physical abilities *doing* tasks become easier.

With movement, the *knowledge* is information about the movement system and the *doing* is practicing moving well. The goal is to get into the Easy/Simple area of the diagram where movement decisions can be made quickly (because of your understanding of how the body works) and easily (as you learn to move your body safely and efficiently – the way it was meant to move). In the Easy/Simple quadrant, movement is a fun and happy experience. Success!

The following examples of a soccer player and a person who has had a knee joint replacement show how a movement of getting from Point A to Point B may be in any of the four quadrants of the Knowing / Doing graphic. In movement, a person's physical abilities and limitations and goals may make a task easy or difficult. The environment may make the task simple or complex.

Soccer player:

Upper right: having no injury and running across a level gym floor kicking a soccer ball is easy and simple.

Lower right: having a sprained ankle makes it difficult, but simple to run across the gym floor kicking a soccer ball.

Upper left: running down a soccer field kicking a ball is easy, but it gets complex when your opponents are trying to stop you from getting down the field, there are divots in the turf, and the sun has gone down.

Lower left: running down a soccer field kicking a ball and you have a sprained ankle and your opponents are trying to stop you from getting down the field, the sun has gone down, and there are divots in the turf, is difficult and complex.

Person with a knee joint replacement:

Upper right: walking to the bathroom with a walker to brush your teeth is simple and easy.

Lower right: walking to the bathroom with a walker and your knee is stiff from swelling, is difficult but simple.

Upper left: walking to the bathroom with a walker is easy but complex when you need to step around or over socks and shoes and the door won't open all the way because it is stuck on a rug.

Lower left: walking to the bathroom with a walker and your knee is stiff from swelling and you need to step around or over socks and shoes, and the bathroom door won't open all the way because it is stuck on a rug is difficult and complex.

The Knowing / Doing graphic also explains how injury may occur during movement. Walking up steps that are perfectly smooth with a sturdy rail presents a lower risk of injury compared to walking up steps that have chunks of concrete missing and a loose rail. The shoes you are wearing, your age, and the weather all add difficulty and complexity to the task. Chapter 28 presents ways to be prepared for movement to lessen the risk for injury.

Using the car analogy, when getting your car inspected, you may be told that your car won't pass unless you spend $1200 to fix the braking system. Hopefully, you were prepared for this unexpected situation and have money in the bank. In the movement world, your 'money in the bank' is extra flexibility, strength, muscle endurance, movement memory (Chapter 17), etc. that you may use when you are faced with unexpected movement demands. Parents teach their children to save money for a rainy day. Healthcare providers encourage movement because we see the people who have had life-changing events due to a fall that occurred because of poor flexibility or being unable to adapt to a movement challenge.

Movement may be difficult and complex for many reasons. As a physical therapist, I have seen a lot of them:

- weakness and low muscle endurance from a previous injury
- range of motion limitations
- time constraints
- sedentary lifestyle
- poor movement training
- poor risk-taking behaviors
- poorly designed work environments or processes

Success in movement is more likely when you identify the obstacles or barriers to movement and figure out how to overcome them. Sometimes the barriers are injuries which happened a long time ago which have been forgotten. In particular, many people don't remember injuring their feet, and they are surprised that something that occurred a long time ago may be contributing to the current pain in their knee, hip, or back. The body's memory of an injury may interfere with current movements. More on how old injuries impact movement in the discussion on compensation (Chapter 16).

So that you and I are moving in the same direction, I want to restate the purpose of this book: to increase your knowledge and understanding of movement to help you move better. A process for lasting improvement in movement is to identify the *cause* of pain or poor performance, treat the *cause*, then restore the flexibility, strength, endurance, etc., and fundamentals of movement (Chapter 25) that are necessary to meet the movement goal.

Where do you stand on the Knowing / Doing graph? The goal is to move from a condition of complex and difficult to where movement is simple and easy.

As a new parent, I often wished our first baby came with a book on what to do when a child is teething, how to teach safety without compromising curiosity, how to know when a rash is serious, etc. My goal is that the information presented in this book will help you to take care of your movement system and make wise movement decisions.

What Happens Next?

Chapter 9 compares the human body to a car. Just like there are many parts of a car that work together to get you from place to place, there are many parts of your body that work together to achieve a desired movement, such as walking up a ramp or reaching down to put water in your dog's bowl. You may realize that you know more about taking care of the parts of your car than you do about the parts of your body. You might be able to buy a new car, but you only get one body. Performing preventative maintenance of the body is a good strategy for moving well from day one of your life to year 101.

Chapter 10 presents information on the names and functions of parts of the body that are used for safe, efficient, pain-free movement. Even if you are knowledgeable on anatomy, please read this chapter as it explains how body parts are meant to be used and, more importantly, how body parts should not be used. For the architects and engineers reading this book, this is a 'form versus function' discussion. Form dictates function or maybe the function modified the form. The chicken or the egg. In either case, body parts are best used in a way that is consistent with their form. If body parts are used to perform a function that they were not meant for, you may experience pain or you may damage the part.

Chapter 11 defines movement terms and explains how some special body parts help to make movement safer and more efficient.

Chapter 12 defines the words safe, efficient, pain-free.

Chapters 13 explains how the brain interprets pain. Pain is a message from the body to the brain. Don't 'kill the messenger (the body)' by ignoring pain.

Chapter 14 discusses muscle inhibition and 'functional weakness.'

Chapter 15 discusses gaining from pain.

Chapter 16 is about compensation, which is what may happen when the body tries to avoid the experience of pain by using another body part to perform a movement. For better performance with less pain, it is a good idea to put the brakes on the compensation – overload – pain – compensation cycle. For teachers of movement (personal trainers, coaches, parents, healthcare providers, teammates, colleagues, etc.), understanding compensation in movement may help to guide training, improve performance, and prevent injury.

Chapter 17 is about how movement involves all of you – physical, emotional, cognitive, and spiritual.

Chapter 18 reminds you that keeping all parts working well maximizes your options for movement.

Chapter 19 explains what is going on behind the scenes in your body when you move.

Chapter 20 presents some misconceptions that you may have about the movement system.

Chapter 21 presents some ideas on preventative maintenance for your body.

Chapter 22 presents what happens normally with aging.

Chapter 23 presents how to document your movement history.

Get to know your body and how it works. Think prevention. Enjoy your ride for a lifetime!

CHAPTER 9

Your Body: Not Just Smart, but 'Genius'

Your body is your car, your vehicle, your way of getting around and enjoying life. Without you taking a class or watching a video, your body knows how to keep you moving after you injure it. In other words, your body knows how to compensate to help you meet your movement goals. That is how smart your body is. But if you make it compensate too much, it may talk to you and the message is pain. If you don't listen, to your body, it may shut you down. Much more on all this later. Let's get into the car – human body analogy.

You want to buy a vehicle. For what purpose? To get to your job? For pleasure? Do you want it to be comfortable for long rides or is it a vehicle meant for short distances? How long do you want to keep it? How many miles do you plan on driving it? Do you want it to purr like a kitten or are you willing to accept squeals and grunts and a not-so-smooth ride?

Is your body just for basic activities like going to work, shopping, and making your bed? Or do you want to navigate creeks and piles of rocks to get a better view, do home-improvement, take care of Mom or Grandma, or live on your own into your 90s? Do you want to be able to dance at a wedding without being laid up the next day, get up and down the basement stairs, or go on a bike ride with your children?

Let's see how owning a car is like owning your body.

What's involved in owning a car:

1. Review the car's history before buying to see if the car was in an accident.

2. Check the owner's manual that outlines the type of fuel to use, how the electronics work, etc. and the preventative maintenance program.

3. Perform preventative maintenance including oil changes, radiator flushes, and periodic replacement of timing belts/spark plugs, tires, windshield wipers, brakes, head, tail, and signal lights, and other parts.

4. Required to pass an annual state inspection and be insured to stay on the road.

5. Operated by a licensed driver who has passed written and road tests.

6. Follow the rules – stop signs, speed limits, and similar rules – or risk losing driving privileges.

7. Loss of function of parts may require repairing or replacing. Sometimes it is possible to keep driving when some of the parts are not functioning well and at other times the car may be unsafe to drive until it is repaired.

8. An efficient way to fix a car is to do a thorough assessment first, then repair or replace the parts that are not working well.

9. It is usually less costly and inconvenient to fix a small problem when you first find it instead of giving it time to potentially turn into a big problem.

10. For the safety of the driver, it is important to make sure the communication system is working properly which includes the head, tail, and signal lights, the horn, windshield wipers and warning lights such as high temperature, low tire pressure, and low fuel.

11. To get to a destination safely, the driver needs to be able to adapt to new situations such as avoiding an animal in the road or how to take a new route when there is road construction.

12. Aging occurs regardless of how well you take care of the car; rubber gaskets harden, tires lose traction, signal lights fail, and seat covers wear out.

13. There are consequences to neglect. A small crack in the windshield may expand so that you won't be able to see clearly to drive safely.

What's involved in owning your body:

1. There is a documented medical history that includes major health conditions such as diabetes or hypertension and surgeries. Minor injuries such as ankle sprains or falls that do not receive medical attention may not be part of the medical record. Events such as getting a finger squeezed in a car door, having a desk fall on a foot, or experiencing back pain after carrying furniture upstairs, sometimes requires probing to be recalled.

2. The body does not come with an owner's manual that states whether a bug bite may be ignored or if it requires a visit to the emergency department. Is it normal for a 60-year-old to fall once or twice a month or does that require medical consultation?

3. You can engage in a preventative maintenance program for your body.

4. Annual inspections are recommended but not required (medical, vision, dental, and hearing).

5. Education on how the body works and a license to 'drive' are not required.

6. There are consequences for breaking the 'rules of the road' of the body such as lifting more than the body parts are prepared for or taking movement risks like walking barefoot on gravel. A warning sign or 'ticket' for a movement error might be pain, injury, or loss of function. You may choose to 'tear up the ticket' by taking a pain medication or compensating with another body part. If you get too many 'tickets', you may lose your ability to meet your movement goals or you may get pain when you do move.

7. Like a car, there is a legal requirement to have insurance to cover costs due to illness or injury.

8. Like a car, there are a lot of parts that work together to cause movement. Sometimes it is possible to keep moving when parts are not functioning well and other times it is not possible.

9. Like a car, the most efficient way to fix the body is to do a thorough assessment first, then treat or replace the parts that are not working well. Pain medications offer temporary relief but may have negative consequences if overused. While replacing worn

parts in a car usually has good results, this may not so true with the body. Surgery itself causes trauma to the body, which may lower movement capabilities.

10. Like a car, it is usually less costly to fix a small problem in terms of time, cost, and pain when first identified instead of waiting until it potentially turns into a big problem.

11. Like a car, for safety, it is important to make sure the sensors are working well such as vision and hearing and using footwear that can sense the surface well.

12. Like the driver of a car, it is good to be able to adapt to new situations such as moving safely and efficiently after a heart attack or toe fracture.

13. Like a car, normal aging of body parts occurs over time. Muscles typically get weaker and less flexible. Vision, hearing, and sense of touch tend to decline.

14. Like a car, there are consequences for neglecting parts such as experiencing back pain from compensating for a knee injury that did not receive proper rehabilitation.

Your body just like your car may perform better if you become knowledgeable about its parts and learn when to seek expert advice. Doing good preventative maintenance for your body and your car may help improve your 'driving' experiences.

Car Analogy

A car's most important function is to get you from Point A to Point B safely. Table 2 lists the analogies between the systems of a car and the systems of the body.

Two body systems that do not have analogies with a car are reproductive and lymphatic. It would be nice (and cheaper) if a car could reproduce and make another car when you want one. A car also doesn't have an immune system. When a car is 'sick,' a mechanic performs diagnostic testing and analyzes information from sensors to locate the problem. This is like a healthcare provider ordering blood work, imaging, and other tests to diagnose your body's sickness.

Table 2: Car – Body Analogies of Systems

Car	Body
Car body	Integumentary — skin
Car frame, chassis	Skeletal
Drive shaft, linkages to wheels	Muscular
Temperature and fuel sensors, wiring, etc.	Sensors, nerves
Engine	Cardiovascular
Carburetor, air filter	Respiratory
Electronic control units	Endocrine
Gas tank, spark plugs, air lines	Digestive
Catalytic converter, exhaust system, oil filter	Urinary, kidney
No analogy	Reproductive
No analogy	Lymphatic
Driver	Brain

What makes your body not just smart, but 'genius,' is its ability to repair itself, such as overcoming viruses and healing skin abrasions and knee sprains. When something is not working in a car like a leaky brake line or a burnt-out headlight, it might be possible to keep driving but it might be risky. In the musculoskeletal system, when a part is not working, the body may compensate by using different muscles and joints to keep the movement going. However, in the body there may be a cost to compensating and it may keep adding up the more you do it. It is good to be the owner of a 'genius car' that has the ability to adapt when parts lose function because unless there is a catastrophic injury, it is usually possible to get your body to a 'repair shop' (residence or a healthcare provider's office) safely without needing to get towed (an ambulance to a hospital). However, like anything else, too much of a good thing – compensating – may be costly in the long run. More on this in Chapter 16.

The heart of the car, the engine, is connected to the drive train and eventually the tires which rotate causing the car to move. The engine relies on the oil pump, lines, and filters to keeps the engine cool, parts lubricated, and to remove impurities. The same functions are needed by the body. The cardiovascular system includes the heart, arteries, and veins. It supplies oxygen, nutrition, and removes waste products. The kidneys play a role in hydration to improve the efficiency of the body like a catalytic converter helps a car to run more efficiently. Hydration, or water content is important for the ability of muscles to contract smoothly with good strength and endurance without going into spasm.

Older cars should be driven regularly to maintain performance and to check for possible deterioration. The same strategy applies to the body. When there are signs of malfunction or weakness, the car or body should be evaluated by someone knowledgeable before taking it 'on the road' that is, doing strenuous activity. In the body, the ability to move may be impaired by deficits in a part, pain, and even the anticipation of pain. Just like a car needs to have its bearings lubricated, the body's muscles and joints need to maintain proper hydration to generate a muscle force and for flexibility and mobility. Movement also may have the effects of stimulating the brain to increase alertness, improve cognitive function and emotional mood, and improve pain tolerance. In sum, when the body moves there is potential to increase 'money in the bank' physically, emotionally, and cognitively.

Becoming more knowledgeable about how the body works is a good way to try to avoid a big repair bill (pain), time lost due to not being able to move, or losing some function altogether. Patients motivated me to write this book because they wanted people to learn from their poor movement choices or the results of unexpected movement challenges. For the entertainment of readers who know a lot more about cars than I do, I'll share some car stories about what I learned through experience rather than reading about cars or learning from experts.

Car Stories and Body Analogies

Car Story A: There are small metal pieces that are precisely placed on wheel rims that make tires balanced so they rotate smoothly. If the pieces fall off or are not put on correctly, the ride may be rough (as mine was). It is inexpensive to get the pieces replaced, and the ride, in my case, was much smoother. With my first new car, I thought the rough ride was the car breaking itself in until I was told that the steering wheel shouldn't vibrate when you go 60 miles per hour.

Body Analogy A: Ideally, new shoes should be comfortable the first time they are worn. 'Breaking in' shoes sometimes means 'breaking in' your feet.

Car Story B: If spark plugs are not gapped correctly, the engine may run rough. Simply gapping the spark plugs correctly may help to avoid a major engine bill. Don't assume anything, even simple things.

Body Analogy B: It's a good idea to stretch muscles and move joints so they are well-prepared for the challenges of a race.

Car Story C: When my car was four years old it was in a minor accident. After the repair, the car handled well for many years. One day when I was driving, I felt a very slight pull of the steering wheel to the left. I thought this might have been due to the road surface. When it happened on another occasion, I decided it was time to seek professional advice.

Body Analogy C: An 8-year-old sprained their ankle while playing soccer. After the pain went away, there were no apparent deficits in movement, and they returned to playing soccer. As a 20-year-old, the same person was experiencing back pain for a day or two after strenuous workouts, so they accommodated by reducing the intensity of their activities. Then one day, they almost fell because they mis-stepped when they were helping someone move a couch. So, they avoided moving heavy furniture and sought professional guidance to address their movement concerns.

Car Story D: If the lug nuts that keep the tires on the car are not tightened well, the car may shake, and it may feel like the car is going to fall apart.

Body Analogy D: If something in your body feels wrong, consider stopping, and checking it out before there is a catastrophe.

What is the take-home message of **A**, **B**, **C**, and **D** from above? Take care of your body like you take care of your car.

A. When engaging in a new movement activity get informed on what to expect.

B. Prepare for movement before moving.

C. Getting older means things are likely going to change. Listen to your body. Get advice on what you may be able to do to continue to move well. Avoid taking unnecessary movement risks.

D. If a movement feels unsafe, stop, and get checked out by a professional.

All body systems play a role in movement. This book focuses on the ones that directly are responsible for movement: skeletal, muscular, and nervous.

1. Skeletal system – bones and joints: framework for the body, protection for vital organs.

2. Muscular system – muscles, tendons, and ligaments: cause body parts to move or stay in one place.

3. Nervous system – sensors, nerves, brain: a) sensors located throughout the body sense pain, touch, stretching, body position and movement, b) nerves like electrical wires send information into, around, and out of the brain, and c) the brain, the car's computer, receives and organizes information from the body, stores memory, develops a movement plan, and activates muscles for coordinated movement.

In any organization, a key to success is communication. The same is true for the body. Table 3 lists the car/body analogies involved in communication.

Table 3: Car – Body Analogies for Communication

Car	Body
Tires	Feet/footwear
Headlights	Eyes
Windshield wipers	Eyelids
Horn	Vocal cords, ears
Fuel gauge, tire pressure and sensors	Pain, muscle, tendon, ligament, joint sensors
Speedometer	Heart/heart rate
Electrical wires	Nerves
Steering wheel/driver	Brain

To promote longevity and comfort, cars and bodies have some added features as listed in Table 4.

Table 4: Car – Body Analogies of Special Parts

Car	Body
Rubber gaskets on oil pan	Meniscus at the knee
Shock absorbers	Intervertebral disks
Cushioned seats	Bursae at hips, knees, shoulders, etc.

CHAPTER 10

Getting to Know Your Body's Parts and Functions

The most important function of the body is to stay alive. To survive, we need to find and get food, run away from danger, and make and use tools to create a safe living environment. To do this we use the five senses that we learned in kindergarten: vision, hearing, smell, taste, and touch. Particularly important for movement and balance are the vision, vestibular, proprioceptive (body awareness), and tactile sensors (Chapter 30). Altogether, the sense of touch provides the brain with information on body position, alignment of body parts, movement, and how we are connected to the environment (standing on a level sidewalk versus a slippery, sloped driveway). How all the senses work together for balance is presented in Chapter 30.

To move safely, efficiently, and pain-free, it is good to know how the size and shape of body parts make them good for some tasks and how they may be harmed if they are doing tasks that they are not meant to do. It's about using the right tool (body part) for the right job.

Stop reading for a minute and look at the skeleton photos in Figures 2, 3, and 4. What were your first observations? Did you wonder why the bones have different shapes and sizes? Did you see anything that surprised you?

As a physical therapist for thirty plus years treating movement problems, I still am amazed at the complexity of the body, and its ability to continue to move even when some parts are not functioning well.

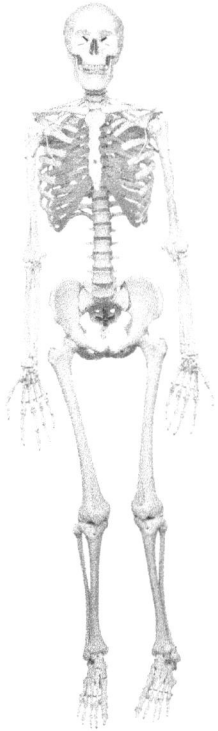 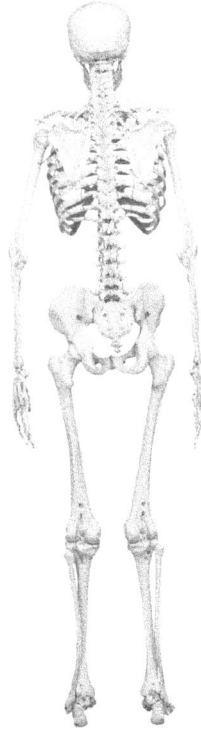 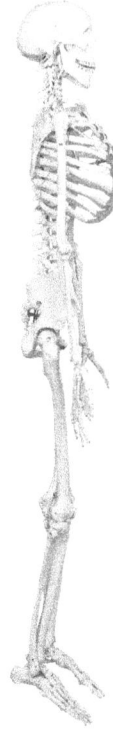

Figure 2	Figure 3	Figure 4

Here is what I see:

- ► There are a lot of bones and joints and they come in a variety of different sizes and shapes.
- ► It looks like the head has a lot of freedom to move compared to other body parts.
- ► The low back area seems unprotected compared to the upper trunk that has a lot of rib bones.
- ► The hip joints look more stable than the shoulder joints.
- ► The feet seem too delicate to support and balance the weight of the body.
- ► The hands and feet look very similar.
- ► It is amazing that so many body parts work together without me having to think about bending my hips and knees, putting weight on the front part of my foot, and reaching out with my hands to take towels out of the dryer.

Body parts have specific functions[17]:

The head contains important organs to sense the environment – eyes, ears, nose, and mouth.

The trunk protects the body's internal organs and provides a safe pathway for the spinal cord.

The upper extremities – shoulders, elbows, wrists, and hands – are light for quick movements. Arm bones are long for reaching and have a lot of joints to allow for a variety of movements like reaching and manipulating objects. The upper extremities may also be used when falling to help prevent the head from hitting the ground.

The lower extremities – hips, knees, ankles, and feet – are larger and heavier than the upper extremities, since they function to support weight in standing and moving.

Leg bones are long to increase height and step length, and the feet have a lot of joints to help maintain balance on uneven surfaces.

The following sections list specific information about the bones and joints of the body. This is some of the information that my patients wished they knew so they didn't have to be my patients – how the body parts are meant to function and how to be careful when using them to minimize injury. Look at the skeleton photos frequently as you read. Your brain stores a lot of information visually – a picture is worth a thousand words.

Before we move on, I will define some medical words that may come up in conversations with healthcare providers and movement instructors. First, what is a joint? A joint is where two bones meet up and movement occurs. The amount of movement at a joint depends on the shape of the bones. There are specific words that are used to describe joint motions that I list below.

Types of Joint Motions

Flexion: bending so that the space between bones becomes smaller like bending your elbow so you can put food into your mouth. Head, neck, and spine flexion means bending forwards such as when looking down to check that your toes are behind the line at the start of a race.

Extension: bending so that the space between bones becomes larger like straightening your elbow when you reach out to shake someone's hand. Head, neck, and spine extension means bending backwards such as when you look at something directly over your head.

Side bending refers to the head and spine: sideways bending of the head, neck, and spine such as when facing a bookshelf, you tilt your head so you can read the title of a book.

Abduction and adduction: movement of a bone away from and closer to the midline of the body, or at the foot and hand, sideways movement away from and closer to the second toe or the third finger.

Rotation: turning the head, neck, and spine to the left and right or turning the hips and shoulders inward or outward from the midline of the body.

The shape of the two bones that make a joint determines what direction the bones can move – flexion/extension, side bending, abduction/adduction, or rotation. A hinge joint like the elbow moves in flexion and extension. The shape of the hip joint allows for motions of flexion/extension, abduction/adduction, and rotation.

As you look at the photos of the joints, you may be able to see why forcing a joint to move in a direction that the bones don't allow may cause an injury. Using joints in the way they were meant to move because of their shape is like driving the right type of vehicle for the intended function. It is appropriate to drive a sedan on open highways to experience a comfortable ride and a truck on gravel back roads where durability is more important.

Body Parts and Their Function

HEAD
Figures 2, 3, 4

Protects the brain and provides a location for the eyes, ears, nose, and mouth to sense the environment.

Head functions: made of several bones connected with suture joints (a special type of joint). Suture joints allow the skull bones to move during childbirth and to grow as an infant's brain develops and grows.

The head is not for: hitting objects repeatedly such as closing a kitchen cabinet.

CERVICAL SPINE (Neck)
Figures 2, 3, 4

Moves the head to gather information from the environment using the eyes, ears, and nose; protects the spinal cord.

Cervical spine functions: can flex and extend, side bend, and rotate.

The cervical spine is not for: holding a phone between the head and shoulder or holding up tiles when installing a ceiling.

THORACIC SPINE/RIBS/BREASTBONE
Figures 2, 3, 4

Protects the heart and lungs, has muscle attachments for breathing, and protects the spinal cord.

Thoracic spine functions: can flex and extend, side bend, and rotate; increases height for an improved view of the surroundings.

Ribs/breastbone (sternum) functions: expand and contract the ribcage when breathing.

The thoracic spine is not for: absorbing force from car accidents, falls, or other activities.

LUMBAR SPINE (Between the thoracic spine and the pelvis)
Figures 2, 3, 4

Protects the spinal cord.

Lumbar spine functions: can flex and extend, side bend, and rotate. The lumbar spine increases height for an improved view of the surroundings.

The lumbar spine is not for: flexing or bending forwards when lifting, which should be done at the hips and knees, or excessive rotation which may overstress the spinal disks.

PELVIS
Figures 5, 6, 7, 8

Supports the upper body and organs, provides space for a fetus to grow and come into the world, and has large areas for attachment of the muscles that connect the upper and lower bodies.

Pelvis functions: large surface for sitting, provides stability for the body, and helps to position the upper and lower bodies for reaching and walking.

The pelvis is not for: using the buttocks to push a couch across the room or repeated trauma like bouncing on the buttocks to descend a flight of stairs.

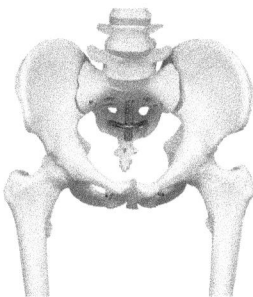 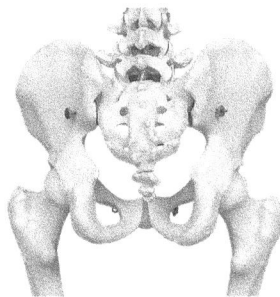 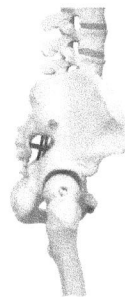 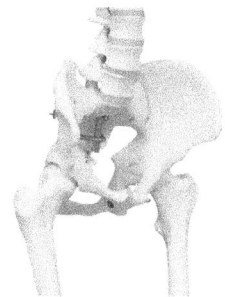

Figure 5   **Figure 6**   **Figure 7**   **Figure 8**

HIP

Figures 5, 6, 7, 8

For walking, running, sitting, bending, and supporting the weight of the body.

Hip functions: can flex and extend, abduct and adduct, and rotate and is a stable joint for transferring weight between the upper and lower bodies.

The hip is not for: letting doors slam on the side of the hip, repetitive fine adjustments for balance when standing on one leg (a task meant for the feet and ankles).

KNEE

Figures 9, 10, 11

For walking, running, shock absorption, and to increase and decrease the height of the body.

Knee functions: can flex and extend, and rotate and is a stable joint for transferring weight.

The knee is not for: kneeling for prolonged times, banging on the kneecap (patella) to close drawers, move boxes, or land from a fall, or excessive twisting when the foot is in a fixed position like in a ski boot.

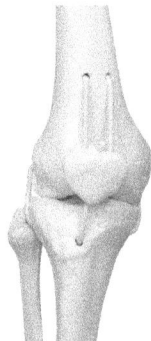 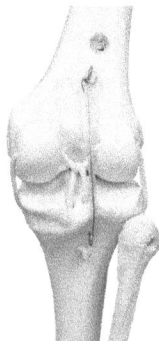 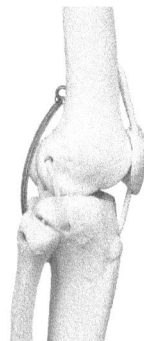

Figure 9   **Figure 10**   **Figure 11**

ANKLE
Figures 12, 13, 14, 15, 16

For squatting, walking, running, and raising body height by going up on tiptoes.

Ankle functions: can flex and extend and is a stable joint for transferring weight.

The ankle is not for: overstretching the ligaments on the lateral (outside) ankle which may cause a sprain such as when landing on someone's foot after getting a rebound in basketball.

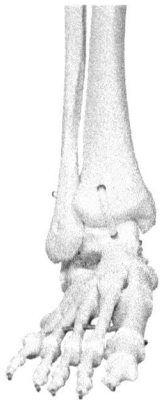
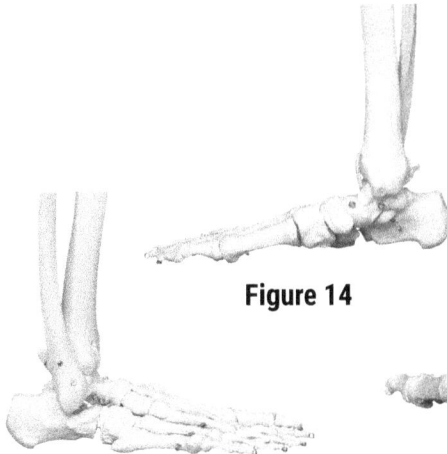
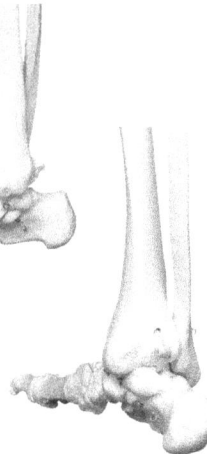
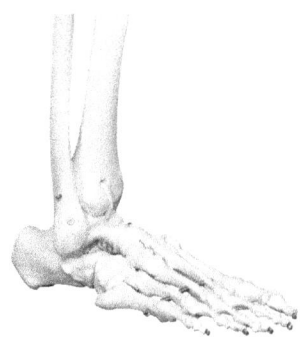

Figure 14

Figure 16

Figure 12

Figure 13

Figure 15

FEET
Figures 17, 18

Sense the ground, perform adjustments for balance, and form a large platform to stand on. For shock absorption, to transfer weight and to provide a direction for movement. The larger bones at the back part of the foot are for bearing weight. The smaller bones in the middle and front of the foot help to accommodate to uneven surfaces. Toes are for weight shifting and balancing (see Chapter 25).

Feet functions: can pronate (flattening of the inner arch) and supinate (raising of the inner arch), and the toes can flex and extend and abduct and adduct. The foot has many joints, muscles, and sensors for controlling balance, arches for stability, pads to cushion loading, and is lightweight for quick movements.

The feet are not for: saving objects from hitting the floor (a shampoo bottle in the shower or a wrench falling off a workbench), kicking tires, boxes, or garbage cans, lifting and positioning plywood for nailing; being stepped on by large dogs or high-heeled shoes while dancing, being rolled over by a stroller or a car, or used as a wedge to hold a door open. The foot is challenged to perform its functions in certain types of footwear particularly flip flops, open-backed sandals, and clogs. To be consistent with the way the foot functions, ideally shoes should support the back of the foot and have ample width in the front of the shoe so the long foot bones are not being squeezed and the toes have some space for mobility. When there is poor heel support, the toes may be busy gripping to keep a shoe from falling off rather than making fine adjustments needed for balance.

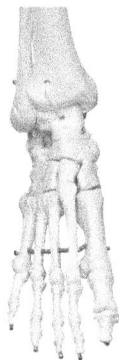 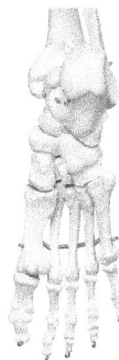

Figure 17   **Figure 18**

SHOULDER
Figures 19, 20, 21, 22

For range of motion and to position the hand.

Shoulder functions: can flex and extend, abduct and adduct, and rotate; a mobile, relatively unstable joint. The shoulder is made up of four joints collectively called a shoulder girdle: (A) the attachment of the shoulder blade to the arm (scapula to humerus – glenohumeral joint, which is what people usually think of when they think of the shoulder joint), (B) the shoulder blade to the trunk (scapulothoracic joint), (C) the collar bone to the shoulder blade (clavicle to scapula – acromioclavicular joint), and (D) the collar bone to the breastbone (clavicle to sternum – sternoclavicular joint). At different times during a movement, each of these four joints needs to be stable or mobile. This requires precise muscle coordination for performing activities such as reaching, dressing, and carrying objects.

The shoulder is not for: weight bearing such as leaning into a refrigerator to move it across the room, carrying heavy objects when the hand is far away from the body, and excessive forces such as when the wind unexpectedly pulls open a door quickly when you are holding it with your hand.

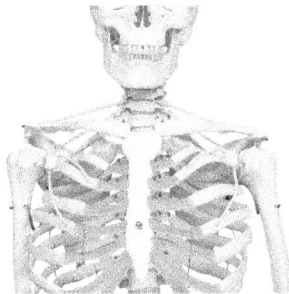

Figure 19

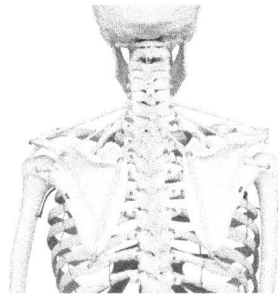

Figure 20

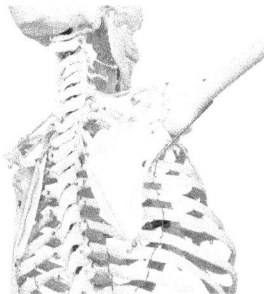

Figure 21

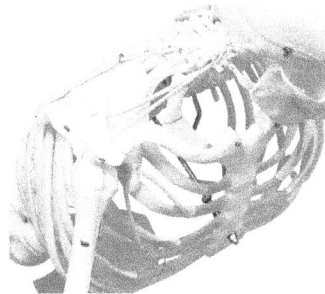

Figure 22

ELBOW AND FOREARM

Figures 23, 24, 25, 26, 27, 28, 29

To lengthen or shorten reach and to position the hand.

Elbow functions: can flex and extend.

Forearm functions: turns palm up (supinates) and down (pronates).

The elbow and forearm are not for: banging the back of the elbow to close a stuck drawer when your hands are full or using the forearm to keep an elevator or subway door from closing.

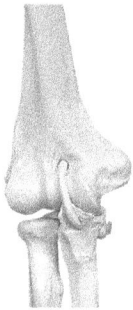 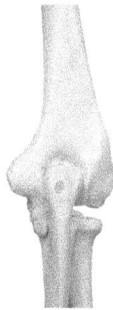 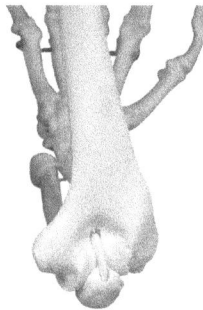 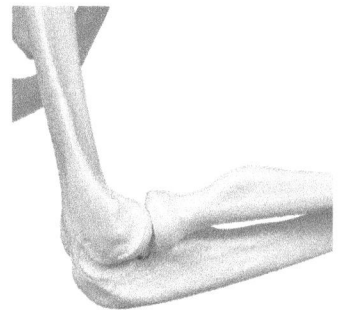

Figure 23   **Figure 24**   **Figure 25**   **Figure 26**

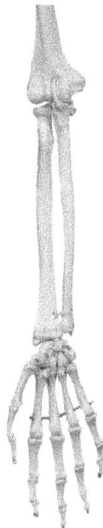 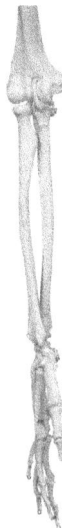 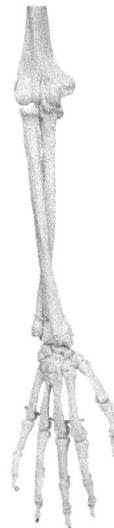

Figure 27   **Figure 28**   **Figure 29**

WRIST
Figures 30, 31

To position and to provide stability for the hand.

Wrist functions: can flex and extend and side bend towards the thumb (radial deviation) and towards the little finger (ulnar deviation).

The wrist is not for: weight bearing when fully extended for prolonged times, such as leaning on a wrist with the palm on the ground when on all fours while gardening.

HAND
Figures 30, 31

For sensing and grasping and manipulating objects.

Hand functions: many sensors, joints, and muscles for precise control of movement, able to adapt to hold objects of different sizes and shapes and are lightweight for quick movements.

The hands are not for: banging on hard surfaces (accidentally hitting the back of your hand when you walk too close to a desk or dresser), carrying heavy objects like a gallon of milk with two fingers rather than your whole hand, or repetitive forceful loading like ripping out shrubs instead of using tools to cut the branches and dig out the roots.

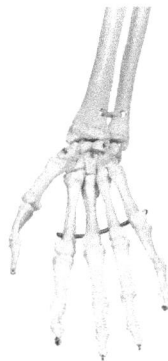 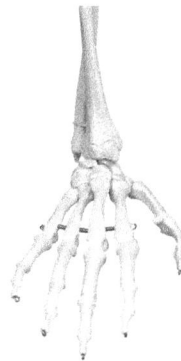

Figure 30   **Figure 31**

CHAPTER 11

Body Language and Special Body Parts

Body Language

Flexibility: ability of skin, muscle, tendons, ligaments, and other soft tissue to get longer or stretch

Mobility: ability of a joint to have a motion; the amount of motion is called the joint's range of motion.

Stability: ability of a joint to stay in one place; a joint may be stabilized by ligaments, tendons, or muscles or by the shape of the bones themselves.

Force: a push or a pull to cause movement or to resist being moved. A force is described in three ways: where the force is being applied, the direction of the force, and the amount of the force that is being applied. For example, opening a door is easiest and most efficient if a large push is applied far away from the hinges, in a direction perpendicular or at right angles to the door. Chapter 16 on compensation discusses forces and force application.

Strength: ability of a muscle to generate a force to keep a joint in one place, to move it, or to control it as it is being moved (controlled bending of the legs when lowering to a squat position).

Endurance: ability of a muscle to continue to generate a force for an extended time.

Power: the combination of force of a muscle and how fast the force can be generated.

Pressure: force over a surface area; pressure is high when a force is applied over a small area and low when a force is applied over a large area.

Ligament: attaches bone to bone, very strong to resist movement, can stretch but cannot actively shorten like a muscle.

Tendon: attaches muscle to bone, can stretch and recoil after being stretched but cannot actively shorten like a muscle.

Muscle: attaches bone to bone via tendons, can shorten (concentric contraction), lengthen (eccentric contraction) or stay at one length to stabilize a joint (isometric contraction).

Special Body Parts

In addition to bones, muscles, tendons, and ligaments there are some special body parts that improve the safety and the efficiency of movement. They are cartilage and bursa.

CARTILAGE

Cartilage: examples of cartilage are the disks in the spine called intervertebral disks, menisci (plural of meniscus) in the knee, and the thin material on the surface of bones where two bones meet to make a joint (articular cartilage). Cartilage functions to lubricate joints, dampen compressive forces and increase the contact area of two bones where they form a joint. A larger contact area means less pressure on tissue since the force is spread over a bigger area. Lower pressures are safer for tissue health whereas higher pressures may lead to injury.

Intervertebral Disks: cartilage between bones of the spine that allow for more range of motion of the spine.

> *Disk characteristics*: disk height is reduced slightly as the day progresses and with increasing age.

Knee Meniscus: cartilage between the thigh bone (femur) and leg bone (tibia) that increases the contact area of the joint. Car analogy: rubber gaskets or washers placed between two metal surfaces.

> *Meniscus function*: crescent-shaped wedge that increases joint contact area.

Articular Cartilage: protects the surfaces of bones where they meet to form a joint.

Articular cartilage characteristic: may be damaged with large loads leading to inflammation (arthritis).

Articular Cartilage is not for: high impact loading like falling or sports-related injuries.

BURSAE

Bursae: fluid-filled sacs that reduce friction and provide a cushion between bones and soft tissue such as tendons and skin. There are many bursae in the body. Bursae that commonly get overloaded, inflamed, and painful are the ones located at the pelvis, hip, knee, and shoulder.

Ischiogluteal Bursa: protects the gluteus maximus at the pelvis.

Ischiogluteal bursa characteristics: sac of fluid may become inflamed with trauma or repetitive loading.

Ischiogluteal bursa is not for: prolonged sitting on hard surfaces.

Greater Trochanter Bursa: protects the soft tissue from rubbing on the greater trochanter of the thigh bone (femur). The greater trochanter is the most lateral part of the femur near the hip joint.

Greater trochanter bursa characteristics: sac of fluid may become inflamed with trauma or repetitive loading.

Greater trochanter bursa is not for: repetitive trauma such as letting a door bang on the greater trochanter or spending long periods of time lying on one side which may cause pain both on the underneath and top greater trochanter areas from pressure, or tension of soft tissue compressing the bursa respectively.

Infrapatellar Bursa: protects the patellar tendon, which connects the kneecap (patella) to the lower leg bone (tibia).

Infrapatellar bursa characteristics: sac of fluid may become inflamed with trauma or repetitive loading.

Infrapatellar bursa is not for: prolonged kneeling on hard surfaces.

Subacromial Bursa: protects part of the rotator cuff at the shoulder.

Subacromial bursa characteristics: sac of fluid may become inflamed with trauma or repetitive loading.

Subacromial bursa is not for: prolonged reaching overhead, sleeping on the stomach with the hand or forearm placed under the head.

CHAPTER 12

The Goal: Safe, Efficient, Pain-Free Movement

Restoring movement abilities and training for higher performance of movement has been my world for more than three decades. Early in my career I was introduced to spinal stabilization training which promotes using the core or abdominal muscles to maintain good postural alignment while restoring movement.[18] There are many other programs to improve movement which typically have the goals of achieving safe, efficient, and pain-free movement. The following definitions describe these three criteria for successful movement.

Safe means very low chance of injury due to loading parts too early, too long, too late, too quickly, or with too much force. An example of safe movement is getting close to an object and lifting with the legs rather than bending at the waist which may potentially overload and cause injury to back muscles.

Efficient means to have maximum productivity with minimum wasted effort. In the body, efficient means starting from a well-aligned, stable posture and using the body parts in the way that they were meant to be used. Using the right tool for the right job in the right way. It means applying force correctly: correct point of application (using the entire hand to carry a heavy binder rather than using the thumb and fingers to hold the binder on one edge), correct direction (closing a drawer by pushing in the direction of the runners versus trying to force a drawer closed by applying a force at an angle to the runners), or using a force that is too little or too much (misjudging the weight of snow and using a shovel with too much or too little effort). Inefficient movement is undesirable because it may lead to tissue injury. When pushing a child in a swing, it would be efficient to stand behind the swing and use the effort of the legs in combination with the arms. It would be less efficient to push the swing when standing at the side of the swing with the arm extended away from the body.

<u>Pain-free</u> is how the brain wants to be. The goal of the brain is survival, which means being safe and avoiding injury. As the next chapter explains, the brain uses pain as an indicator of the safety of a movement. To protect the body, the brain may choose to modify a movement so it may be done with no or minimal pain. Examples include walking *quickly* on hot sand when barefoot or *suddenly dropping* a heavy suitcase or a weight to help prevent an injury. Since avoiding pain is the priority, the brain may have to compromise efficiency and use an alternate group of muscles and joints to carry out a task. In other words, to be safe and pain-free, the brain may choose to use a compensatory movement strategy.

Knowing that the brain prioritizes avoiding pain, it is essential to listen to, and not ignore pain. As the fox in Antoine de Saint-Exupéry's book *The Little Prince* says, "What is essential is invisible to the eye."[19] Pain is invisible, but it is essential.

CHAPTER 13

Pain Is the Body's Traffic Light

What is pain? Pain is a sensation and a perception. Pain is the body's way of communicating.[13,20] There are at least two reasons why you may be having pain during or after movement. Firstly, it may be that a body part is being overloaded. Secondly, there may be a body part that is compensating and being used beyond its capabilities and may be at risk for injury.

Pain Is a Sensation

Just like touch sensors detect and communicate information to the brain, there are sensors all over the body that tell the brain that something is painful. In an acute injury, pain is experienced as a threat. The body responds to the threat by having a sympathetic response: heart rate and blood pressure increase, and muscles become tense to get ready to get away from what is causing the pain to help prevent further injury.

Pain Is a Perception - Pain Is Subjective

How pain is valued and the response to pain varies with the individual and with the situation. Someone may have a low or high tolerance for pain. A person who has low tolerance for pain may stop an activity when they first sense pain, or move cautiously and stiffly which decreases their ability to adapt to a loss of balance, or they may avoid the activity altogether. A person with a high tolerance for pain may keep doing the activity until the pain reaches a very high level, perhaps after a tissue has already been injured.

Both extremes may result in movement problems in the long term. Avoiding activity may lead to muscle weakness and atrophy from disuse. Continuing to be active when there is a large amount of pain (the no-pain, no-gain philosophy) may result in an injury from overuse and/or muscle stiffening or guarding. Muscle guarding is a protective response of the body. When an injury has occurred, or the brain is in protective mode because of the anticipation of pain, the muscles surrounding the injured area may tighten up to 'guard' the joint. This may prevent a joint from moving, effectively functioning like a brace. Muscle guarding interferes with a muscle's ability to relax, which may lead to a loss of balance or a fall.

The mechanisms involved in the perception of pain are beyond the scope of this book and the reader is referred to other sources.[13,20] Briefly, perception of pain:

A. May vary depending on the emotional state such as feeling fearful, anxious, stressed, or depressed.

B. May be lowered by touch and movement. This may explain the reflexive reaction to rub something that hurts or 'walking it off' after getting kicked in the shin.

C. May be altered by thoughts. Decreasing sensitivity to pain or being able to tolerate pain better, may be achieved by mindfulness and thinking calm and peaceful thoughts.

Using the car analogy, pain is communicated from the body to the brain similar to the way road signs and traffic lights communicate information to the driver. There are many forms of 'stop signs' on the road and in the body. Each has a special meaning resulting in different responses.

Red, Amber, and Green Traffic Lights and Road Signs

- ▶ Red traffic light: stop and wait your turn
- ▶ Amber traffic light: slow down, proceed with caution, and be prepared to stop
- ▶ Green traffic light: keep going and proceed with caution
- ▶ Red stop sign: full stop, look both ways, proceed with caution
- ▶ Triangular amber yield sign: slow down and proceed with caution
- ▶ Construction worker standing with a sign that says 'stop' or 'slow down': stop or slow down and be careful of the road conditions
- ▶ Red flashing lights at railroad crossing: stop, listen, and stay off the track
- ▶ Red flashing lights and stop sign on a school bus: stop, stay back, and look for children

The same color system may be used to explain how pain communicates specific information to the brain. Physical pain may be labeled as acute pain (red), chronic pain (with a subset of 'compensatory pain') (amber), and good pain (green). Each type of pain sends a unique message to the brain which causes a unique response. When the body communicates pain, it might be a threat to survival like red lights flashing at a railroad crossing or something that slows you down temporarily like an amber yield sign.

In sum:

- ▶ Red signals acute pain: stop
- ▶ Amber signals chronic and 'compensatory pain': slow down, assess the situation, be prepared to stop, and proceed with caution
- ▶ Green signals good pain: there is no need for concern; keep driving the car (moving the body)

Red Light: Acute Pain

In the movement system, acute pain happens when there is cell injury due to a mechanical event like tearing a meniscus of the knee or being cut with a piece of glass. Acute pain is felt at a high level and is persistent. The message to the brain in acute pain is, "Stop what you are doing right now and let this heal." In the 'rules of the road' car analogy, acute pain is a red traffic light, a red flashing light at a railroad crossing, or a school bus stop sign with flashing red lights.

Acute Pain and the Inflammatory Process

After an acute injury, the body automatically initiates a three-step process of healing: 1) inflammatory phase, 2) anti-inflammatory / repair phase, and 3) remodeling phase. During the inflammatory phase, chemicals are released and when they contact nerves they communicate 'pain' to the brain. This is 'protective pain.' It tells the person to stop using that body part because it is injured and let it rest so it may heal. Depending on the severity of the trauma – bruising a knee on a drawer versus fracturing a kneecap (patella) from a fall – you may be able to use the knee immediately or in six to eight weeks after the bone has healed.

A closer look at the three-step process of tissue healing:

1. <u>The inflammatory phase (Day 1 to about Day 4-7):</u> "**PRISH**" is the acronym for **P**ain, **R**edness, **I**mmobility, **S**welling, and **H**eat.

   ▶ Changes in blood flow result in **H**eat, **R**edness, **S**welling. The swelling limits the bending at a joint effectively stabilizing the injury to protect it from further injury and to allow healing.
   ▶ Chemicals are released that increase sensitivity to **P**ain. Other cells come in to remove the damaged tissue and debris from the inflammatory process.
   ▶ Pain may lead to a loss of function or **I**mmobility.

2. <u>The anti-inflammatory / repair phase (begins about Day 4 and continues to about 4-6 weeks):</u>

   ▶ New collagen fibers are laid down haphazardly to provide a framework for the next phase of healing.
   ▶ Other cells fill in the framework to help with the repair process.

3. <u>The remodeling phase (from about 2 weeks to over a year):</u>

    ▶ The goal of the remodeling phase is to improve the alignment of collagen fibers and their ability to slide on each other to improve the flexibility and strength of the repair. When remodeling, connections between the fibers may prevent the fibers from sliding on each other easily which may result in scar tissue. This scar tissue may lead to inflexibility and 'functional weakness' which may have a big impact on movement (discussed in Chapter 14).

Amber Light: Chronic Pain

Chronic pain is milder than acute pain, varies in intensity and sometimes may be relieved by resting or changing postures or activities. In chronic pain, the brain may interpret the pain message to mean 'slow down,' because the body is not 'operating on all cylinders' and there may be an increased risk for injury. As with driving, an amber traffic light for the movement system means slow down, proceed with caution, and be prepared to stop. Chronic pain is pain that typically has gone on for at least three months. By this time, testing and assessment to identify the cause of the pain has usually been exhausted. Perhaps the cause of the pain was identified, such as a change in anatomy or irreversible tissue damage where return to normal function may not be expected. Or the precise cause of the pain may not have been identified.

Amber Light: 'Compensatory Pain'

There is another 'amber light' type of pain, that I am going to call 'compensatory pain' for the purposes of discussion in this book. Like chronic pain, compensatory pain is milder than acute pain and it may be relieved by rest. Compensatory pain comes from tissues that are compensating for an injury, a movement deficit, or a movement challenge. For example, if you are limping due to right knee pain, you may be overloading the left hip which is causing compensatory left hip pain. After the right knee pain is gone (perhaps because the knee is not being used much causing it to be weak from disuse), you may still be experiencing left hip pain. A solution to getting rid of the left hip pain might be to strengthen the right knee to decrease the excessive loading on the left hip.

Compensatory pain may be relieved by reducing the overloading of the painful structure which may be done by resting or changing postures or activities. In compensatory pain, the brain receives a message, "You are overloading tissue, and I am at risk for injury." Compensatory pain signals the brain to slow down, assess the situation, be prepared to stop, and proceed with caution. The person with compensatory pain may have the following symptoms.

- ▶ Pain is mild compared to acute pain.
- ▶ Besides pain, there may be other sensations such as aching, sharp, numb, tingling, sore like a bruise, or burning.
- ▶ The sensations may last for a few seconds or for hours and may stop if postures or movements are modified.
- ▶ The sensations may come and go in one or many locations of the body. They may be brief or continue for hours, days or weeks at each location. The symptoms may repeat in cycles in the same locations as the body switches between using and resting compensatory parts.
- ▶ The area of the sensation may be more tender to touch than nearby tissue or the same body part on the opposite side of the body. This tenderness indicates that the tissue is hypersensitive to pain, which may prevent the tissue from functioning normally.
- ▶ The person may change how the activity is performed, try different footwear or equipment, or they may avoid the activity altogether. This is like taking another route to get to work to avoid yield signs.
- ▶ There may be chronic muscle tightness of the muscles that are compensating.

Often it is challenging to identify the *cause* of pain because the pain sensation from the initial injury is not currently present and the original injury may be long forgotten. The brain may now be communicating sensations from compensating tissues. I have yet to hear a patient say, "I broke my little toe at age seven when I jumped off a jungle gym. Can you get my foot working correctly so I can stop having pain in my hip from compensating for my old foot injury?" I hope this puts an end to the question, "What exercise can I do to get rid of the pain in my … (fill in the blank)?"

Green Light: Good Pain

'Good pain' seems to be a contradictory term, but it is often used by patients. When deep pressure is applied to tissue that was injured and has healed, there may be a sensation of 'good pain' which is uncomfortable, yet acceptable, and in fact desirable. Patients say that "this area needs to be touched because I know I will feel better afterwards." With 'good pain,' the body seems to be aware that the uncomfortable sensation is not a threat as in acute pain, and there is no need to withdraw from the touch. They are surprised that with deep pressure, they are sensing pain in a part of their body that is typically pain-free. Patients feel in control of this 'good pain' because they "know the tissue is not being injured and the uncomfortable sensation will stop after the pressure is removed." Perhaps 'good pain' is the body's signal that the healing and recovery process is still in progress and the tissue needs some attention.

Before moving on to the next chapter, have a look at Figure 32, which shows how tissue injury may affect movement if there is pain and development of scar tissue. Immediately after tissue is injured the three-phase healing process begins. To keep you moving, the body may use strategies to avoid the experience of pain – your 'genius car' at work. For example, when a muscle is strained, the brain may select other compensatory muscles to perform the movement. In the case of an injury to a joint, muscles may be used to 'guard' or hold the joint in a fixed position to protect it from further injury, a compensation called 'muscle guarding.' Both strategies allow the injured tissue to rest. For example, if you recently sprained your thumb, you may compensate by tucking your laptop under your arm rather than holding it with your hand as you usually do. A thorough discussion on compensating is presented in Chapter 16.

Besides pain, another effect of an injury may be the development of scar tissue. During phase two of the healing process, collagen fibers are laid down to protect the injured area from further injury and to set up the body for phase three of healing. All these situations – muscle guarding, use of compensatory muscles, and the effects of scar tissue (Chapter 14) – may result in compensatory muscles being overloaded and fatigued. The flowsheet in Figure 32 shows how overused muscles may lead to a cascade of weakness, tightness, and limitations in joint ranges of motion resulting in fewer options for movement. Any of these conditions may increase the risk for more injury.

Figure 32: Tissue Injury and Movement

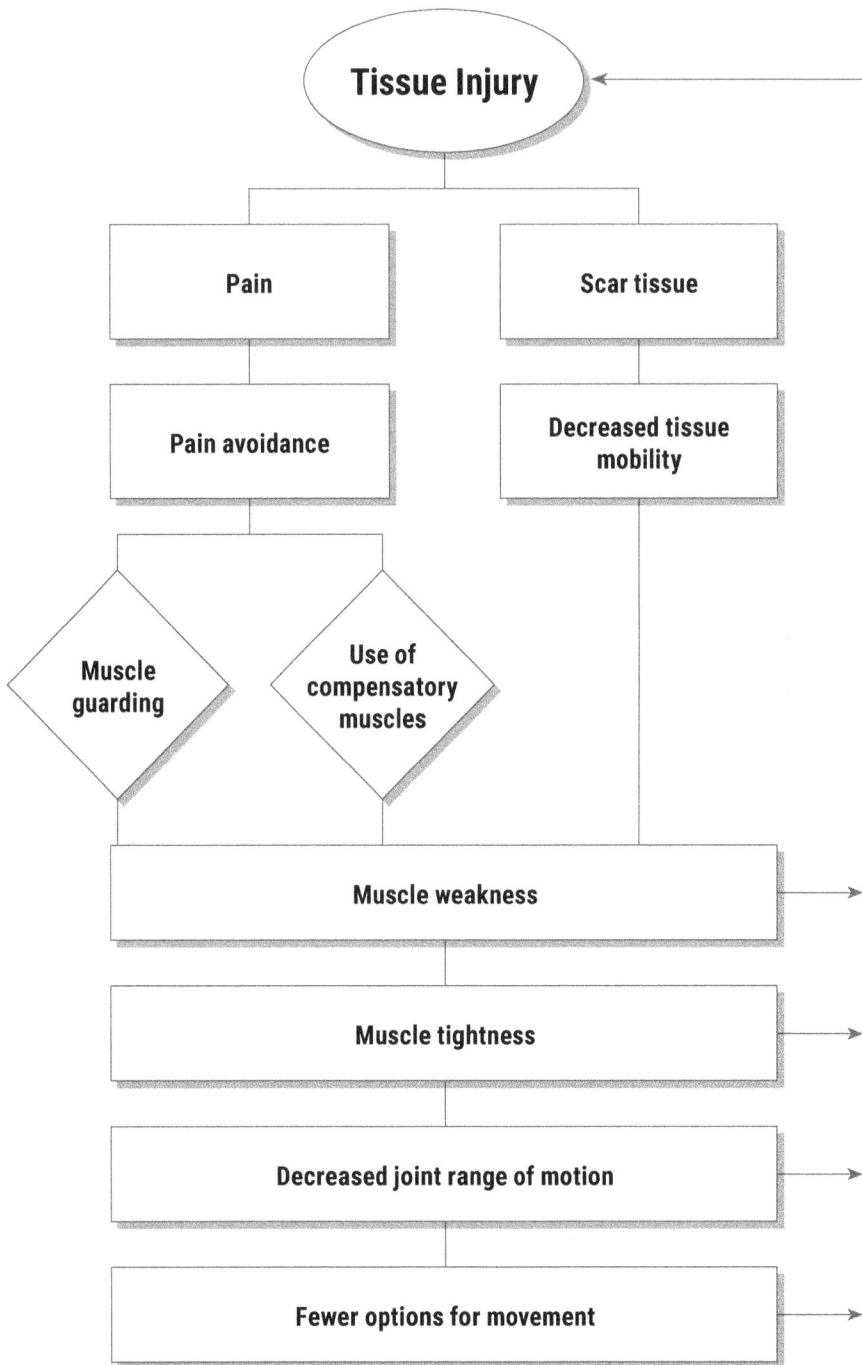

CHAPTER 14

Muscle Inhibition and 'Functional Weakness'

Muscles may be weak or strong, but also may be 'functionally weak' because they are inhibited. This chapter explains why a muscle may be inhibited, how inhibition may lead to 'weakness,' and what may be done to reduce muscle inhibition. A common thought is that a 'weak' muscle needs to be challenged by resistive exercises to get 'stronger.' To solve a 'weakness' problem, it is important to know if a muscle is 'weak' from disuse or if it is 'functionally weak.'

When a muscle is weak from disuse, it might be appropriate to engage in a strengthening exercise program. On the other hand, if a muscle is 'functionally weak' because it is inhibited, a strengthening program may only add to the inhibition. Muscle inhibition refers to a muscle that is lacking the correct signal from the nervous system to function. 'Functional weakness' is a term used in this book to describe a muscle that is functioning weakly due to inhibition.

A muscle may be inhibited because of:

1. Pain[13,21]

2. Swelling around a joint[21]

3. Decreased ability for muscle fibers to slide on each other (scar adhesions)

4. Too much resistance

5. Trigger points which are taut bands in muscles caused by acute or chronic overloading.[22]

Question: *What happens when a muscle is inhibited?*

Answer: When a muscle is inhibited and the movement is continued, other muscles or group of muscles may be activated to compensate.

Question: *How might inhibition of a muscle be lessened?*

Answer: Using a logical argument, perhaps muscle inhibition may be lessened by removing what caused the inhibition. This may be accomplished by decreasing pain, decreasing swelling[21], improving the ability of muscle fibers to slide on each other, decreasing resistance demands, or eliminating trigger points.[22]

Question: *How may pain be decreased?*

Answer: Because pain is a perception, and it varies with the individual and the situation[23] there likely is not one answer on how to decrease pain. From a physical therapy perspective, there is some research evidence that manual therapy decreases pain in people with musculoskeletal disorders.[23] The mechanisms that cause a decrease in pain may be biomechanical, neurophysiological, psychological, or non-specific factors such as patient expectations, client/provider alliance.[23] Regardless of the explanation, manual therapy has been shown to be an intervention that decreases pain. Lessening muscle inhibition due to pain, might be a beneficial strategy to restore muscle 'strength.' You may have used this strategy yourself. Have you ever had a piece of gravel in your shoe that was affecting how you walk? After you removed the gravel that was causing pain (inhibition) and an uneven, unbalanced gait, you immediately walked without compensating. By eliminating the pain from stepping on the gravel or the *anticipation* of pain from possibly stepping on the gravel, you appeared to be functioning 'stronger' as demonstrated by a more even and balanced gait.

Removing inhibition and having an improvement in function is something that we experience in everyday life. How well you sing your favorite song likely depends on your audience. In front of a group, you may be shy and sing softly. You may be reluctant to sing loudly because you fear embarrassment and your singing sounds 'functionally weak.' When you are at home alone and you are not inhibited, you sing 'loudly' with good 'strength.' In the body, fear of pain may be causing a muscle to be 'functionally weak.' When the fear of pain is removed, a muscle may immediately demonstrate 'strength.' If the goal is to be 'strong,' an appropriate intervention may be to find and reduce the inhibition that is causing a muscle to be 'functionally weak' then engage in a strengthening exercise program.

Another cause of 'functional weakness' may be resistance to fibers sliding on each other such as from scar adhesions (see next section). An analogy is pushing a box across a room on a rough surface versus a smooth surface. If you were to push a box of books that is on carpet, you may appear 'functionally weak' because there is a lot of friction, resistance to slide, between the carpet and the box. If you decide to push the same box of books across a wooden floor, it is easier because there is less friction, and you would appear 'stronger.'

Another situation when a muscle may be inhibited is when there is too much resistance and a perceived threat of injury. An analogy for inhibition due to too much resistance is when you try to unzip a zipper that is stuck. If a zipper is difficult to open because a piece of fabric is snagged in the zipper, you may risk breaking the zipper if you use too much force to try to get it to open so you stop trying. The brain prioritizes survival, so if it senses too much resistance, it may stop functioning to avoid injury.

What Is Scar Tissue?

Scar tissue, like lasagna, may be a good thing or a bad thing, depending on the quality and quantity of it. Scarring is good because it protects the tissue that was weakened by injury. However, scar tissue adhesions may become a problem if they interfere with the flexibility of tissue or the ability of a muscle to shorten to generate a force.

Let's take a brief look at how scar tissue develops:

In phase two of tissue healing (about day 4 to about 6 weeks) tissue is repaired by the laying down of collagen fibers in a random fashion. Cells are sent to the injured area to make the fibers stick to each other to improve strength. The combination of the collagen fibers and the cells is called scar tissue. This scar tissue is the body's bandage, which functions to protect the tissue that was injured. Like a bandage, scar tissue connects or adheres to uninjured tissue as well as itself. Hence the term 'scar adhesions.' When there is a large area of tissue injury, there is a need for more 'bandages' possibly leading to more scar adhesions.

How is lasagna like tissue healing? To make lasagna, dry noodles are randomly put in boiling water. After the noodles are cooked and drained (without rinsing them in cold water), the noodles stick to each other because of the starch in the water. This is like tissue healing where starch-like cells stick collagen fibers to each other. The sticky noodles are strong but are limited in their flexibility. To continue making the lasagna, rinse the noodles in cold water so they may easily be separated. Then layer them in a pan in rows with sauce etc.

Scar tissue is three-dimensional like the pot of lasagna noodles. The layers may adhere to each other starting from the surface of the skin down into the body. Muscle fibers also need water to be able to slide on each other when the muscle contracts and to allow stretching when joints are moved (like the lasagna noodles need water so they can be separated easily).

It is possible to palpate (feel) the scar tissue that is formed from surgeries, skin abrasions, and muscle tears. The healing process that occurs in the above situations as well as for tendonitis, bursitis, and arthritis may potentially result in the formation of scar adhesions and the after-effects. The amount of scar tissue and scar adhesions that is formed from the healing process of an injury is an unknown and perhaps varies with the individual. The next section presents how scar tissue and adhesions may be affecting how you move.

Scar Tissue and Movement

Scar tissue may interfere with the flexibility of tissue and strength of a muscle if the fibers are not lined up in the same direction as the tissue or muscle. Manual mobilization of scar tissue may help reduce the potential for adhesions to form so fibers may slide on each other freely. Imagine trying to bend your finger if you don't remove the bandage you placed over a joint when it was initially injured. Just like the bandage on your finger may limit flexibility and mobility, scar tissue may lessen the sliding ability of ligaments, tendons, muscles, and tissues that surround joints. Decreased ability of tissues to slide on each other may lead to a vicious cycle of more injury, inflammation, more scar tissue, decreasing flexibility, and more 'functional weakness.'

Unlike a bandage on your injured finger that can be seen and readily removed, scar tissue under the skin cannot be seen and is usually not painful except when palpated deeply. Just because you can't see or feel scar tissue does not mean that it is not there. The consequences of scar tissue – decreased flexibility and 'functional weakness' – are more obvious. If you had an injury that appears to have healed and is pain-free, you still may have scar tissue that is interfering with your movements. While you may have forgotten about the injury, you may be compensating for flexibility or 'strength' deficits. Compensating may lead to pain in other parts of your body. If you are experiencing a movement problem that seems to be getting better but never really goes away, you may benefit from professional evaluation to determine if you have scar adhesions that may be interfering with your flexibility and/or 'strength.' As with your vehicle, it is usually better to address a small concern before it becomes a bigger problem.

In sum, while tissues may be healed because time has gone by, it does not necessarily mean that their abilities to stretch and/or generate forces have been restored. In the car analogy, a replacement part may not have the same 'abilities' as the original part. Having too many substandard car parts or body injuries that have not been restored to their original level of function may be a recipe for poor performance and/or pain. In the body, 'out of sight' may not mean 'out of mind.' The brain knows about scar adhesions even though they may be out of your sight. Scar tissue and scar adhesions may be interfering with tissue flexibility and 'strength' which may set you up for more injury (Figure 32).

The next chapter combines the knowledge of pain, scar tissue, compensation, and safe and efficient movement to explain how you may be able to gain from pain.

CHAPTER 15

Gaining From Pain:
Be Nice to the Messenger

Recall that pain is the messenger that is used by the body to communicate that you need to do something to keep body parts safe. In all three types of pain mentioned earlier, there is potential for gain. In acute pain, **the gain** may be that when an activity is stopped, further injury may be avoided. In compensatory pain, **the gain** may be that the brain is receiving a message that the body is compensating, and you may benefit from seeking professional guidance to avoid a potential injury. In 'good pain', **the gain** from pain may be that scar tissue has been identified and interventions may been undertaken with the goals of removing inhibitions and improving flexibility and 'strength.'

Identifying old injuries may be challenging because compensatory tissues may be speaking the language of pain and the original injury is not 'talking' at all. Essentially, compensatory pain may be a distraction when trying to find the original injury that is *causing* the compensations. It may be difficult to find the original injury because it is long forgotten, and it is being hidden by layers of compensations.

Here is a process for trying to find the location of old injuries: a) gather information on flexibility, joint range of motion, strength, power, endurance, coordination, and balance, b) have knowledge of all the parts of the movement system and how they work together, c) observe and analyze movements looking for compensations that may be causing tissue overload or disuse, and d) palpate structures that might be contributing to the movement issues to see if there is pain or scar tissue.

Improvement in flexibility, strength, joint range of motion, coordination, and balance may occur following interventions that release scar adhesions and/or reduce pain. When the function of tissue that was previously injured has been restored and is selected by the brain to accomplish a movement, compensations will no longer be necessary. The **gain from pain** that may have been experienced during deep palpation ('good pain') is the restoration of safe, efficient, pain-free movement.

CHAPTER 16

"I Know I Am Compensating"

Why does the body compensate? The body's main goal is to survive so it will do what is necessary to protect itself. From Chapter 13, you learned that pain may be interpreted as a threat to survival – something to fear. The fear-avoidance model of pain is defined as the avoidance of movements based on the fear of anticipated pain. When there is a possibility that a movement may cause pain or injury, the body may come up with a way to move, that is compensate, by using other parts to achieve the movement goal. Typically called fear-avoidance movements, in this book compensatory movements due to fear of pain will be called fear/pain-avoidance movements. This wording is used in discussions on movement when compensations are due to the fear of anticipated pain and not from other sources such as a fear of falling.

Compensating may be a temporary solution to meet your movement goals but that might not work for you in the long term. For example, you may be able to compensate and run one mile without pain, but to get a serotonin jolt by completing a race you need to run three miles.

How Does Compensating Come About?

To compensate means to provide something to make up for a loss or to lessen something that is unpleasant. For example, you may be given a price discount when you buy a table that has a loss in quality because there is a scratch on it. When it comes to pain, compensate means to provide a movement alternative to avoid a known pain. Perhaps you had knee pain when squatting to lift a child out of a stroller, so you changed your lifting technique. You compensated by bending at your back the next two times you lifted a child out of a stroller. However, the third time you used your back to compensate for difficulty squatting, you got back pain. Or, you overdid it at the gym and had thigh pain the next day, so you skipped your next gym session and the pain went away. In these scenarios, compensations temporarily fixed your problem but eventually caused a new problem: back pain or a delay in your strength training because you skipped a gym session.

You know why the body compensates but how does it know when to compensate? The body has a lot of options for movement. Since survival is a primary objective, the brain likely will select the most efficient group of muscles and joints first, which we'll call team A. If the body experiences pain in team A, it may let team A rest and it selects another group of muscles and joints (team B) to perform the movement successfully without pain. This is called a fear/pain-avoidance movement, or compensation, which is the brain's way of protecting tissue and avoiding pain. The muscles and joints on team B may not be as flexible, strong, or coordinated as the ones on team A so they may have an increased risk of injury. The body is getting the job done, but team B is compensating for team A's inability to perform its job.

Team B may continue to function until it gets injured and/or experiences pain, then your brain may call on an even less efficient team C to compensate. Ultimately, compensating for a loss in function might be costly. You may be able to perform a movement, but some parts of your body may be paying a hefty price.

Perhaps you have decided that you are not going to compensate. You are going to work through the pain. You are thinking, "I have a high pain threshold and I can work through the pain. I want to use my injured painful muscle the way it is supposed to be used – the right amount of force at the right time for the right duration." Your brain might be a step ahead of you. Since the brain may be prioritizing survival of body parts over you feeling accomplished by getting through a gym workout, the brain may go into fear/pain-avoidance mode. Pain may inhibit muscle function. If you do try to use team A that is having pain, inhibition from fear/pain-avoidance may result in team B's muscles and joints being called in without you knowing it. I have heard people say, "I know I am compensating because if I don't, I will have pain."

When a frustrated patient comes to me and says, "I have tried everything and I am still not better" I hear, "Can you please find and treat my original injury so I can stop compensating and get permanent relief of this pain?" When someone is having knee pain at age 40, they usually don't remember that they bruised their thigh 100 times when they were a baseball catcher at age 10. You, like other people, may believe that when there is no more pain after an injury and enough time has passed, everything is back to normal. From my experience as a physical therapist, I am going to disagree with you. You may be moving without pain because you have a lot of options to compensate. This may work for you until your options to compensate are used up, you try to improve your movement performance, or when aging takes away some of your options (Chapter 17). Maximizing your options for movement is a topic in Chapter 18.

The take-home message is that compensating for an untreated injury may be a temporary solution. If movement demands increase or the ability to compensate decreases, the brain may send out a pain signal. In a car, a signal might be the 'check engine' light appearing on your dashboard. It is possible to cover the warning sign with a piece of tape but there may be a big price to pay later if the engine seizes up. The same is true for the body.

Let's review what happens after an injury (Chapter 14). In phase one of the healing process, cells are sent to the injured part to protect it from further injury.

In phase two, fibers and other cells are laid down (the body's own bandage) to support the injured tissue. This is called scar tissue. Scar tissue may adhere or stick to any tissue, forming scar adhesions and causing restrictions in nearby, muscles, tendons, etc. Typically, scar tissue is not as flexible or as strong as the original body part. In the car analogy, scar tissue may be like replacing tires with ones that have a lower rating. The 'replacement' scar tissue is not made up of the same type of cells as the damaged tissue therefore does not have the same abilities. For example, scar tissue cannot generate a force like muscle tissue does.

Besides flexibility and strength losses from an injury, there may be losses in sensation. People who have had an ankle sprain demonstrate deficits in the sensations of joint position (proprioception)[24] and vibration.[25] Thus, following an injury, the brain may be getting less sensory information on the position of a joint. Like a GPS, the brain needs to know the position of body parts accurately at the beginning and throughout a movement for you to reach your destination, that is, accomplish the movement goal safely and efficiently. When position information is inaccurate, movement may be less efficient. Less efficient movement may mean more compensations.

Phase three of tissue healing is remodeling where tissue flexibility and 'strength' may improve but not necessarily restored to the pre-injury levels because of scar adhesions. Getting back to teams A, B, and C, when acute pain is gone, the brain may let team A back in the game. Since team A has been out of action, it is likely that full function has not been restored. Team A's muscles may fatigue early, and team B or C may be called in to help. This again may put teams B and C at risk of injury. The compensating teams B and C may get overloaded, get a rest, then get overloaded again. This way of compensating may explain why pain comes and goes in different parts of the body in a familiar cycle.

There is a process for breaking the compensatory pain cycle: find what was injured on team A and work on removing inhibitions that may be interfering with tissue function. You made need professional assistance to identify and improve the flexibility and 'strength' of tissue that was injured considering there may be scar tissue that is interfering with function. The goal is to avoid overstretching normal tissue which may give only temporary improvement in flexibility, joint range of motion, and 'strength.' Treating compensations rather than the *cause* of the movement problem may explain why your muscles feel tight, or your strength just doesn't seem to be coming back the way you think it should.

Let's assume your team A is at full flexibility, strength, and endurance. After sitting on the bench for three weeks because of an injury, the coach (brain) may not let you play (perform the movement). Team B has demonstrated success at winning games without team A and the coach may choose the philosophy, "If it ain't broke, don't fix it." To get called in to play, team A needs to prove to the coach (your brain) that they have restored their ability to move in terms of speed of contraction, timing, sequencing of muscles, endurance, postural alignment and stability, weight shifting, and balance, etc. When the coach (your brain) has replaced their old memories of team A's disabilities with current information of team A's abilities, and the coach has had enough of team B's inadequacies (pain, tightness, weakness), they (your brain) may decide it is safest and most efficient to put team A back in the starting line-up.

Here is another analogy to help you to understand compensation and fear/pain-avoidance movements.

There are many types and sizes of bridges to transport cargo across a river. There are foot bridges made of wood for people, covered bridges made of wood and concrete limited to horses and buggies, suspension bridges for cars and trucks, and even stronger bridges for trains full of heavy cargo. If the suspension bridge is under construction, you may drive your car across the compensatory covered bridge, but that may cause some damage to the bridge making it less usable. It is best to use a bridge or a body part for its intended cargo or function.

In the body there are small muscles and small joints and large muscles and larger joints all for specific purposes. Your goals may be to use your hand and wrist to write a shopping list and to lift a gallon of milk. You need good finger dexterity to write and a strong grasp using wrist muscles to pick up a heavy weight. If your wrist was injured, you may compensate by picking up a gallon of milk by straining small finger muscles. Or if your small finger muscles were injured, you may have poor coordination when you try to write using the strong grasping muscles. Compensating may result in overloading tissue or less than ideal function.

A compensating muscle that performs the function of the injured muscle is likely less efficient than the original muscle because of its anatomical location, muscle size, strength, and endurance. It is like training an employee to use a computer then putting them on the loading dock where they are responsible for unloading trucks. The 'job' of a muscle is determined by its 'line of action of force.' One muscle may be positioned to flex a joint and another muscle may be positioned to cause flexion and side bending at the same time. A muscle is most efficient when the force it generates is in the same direction of the desired movement. If you only want flexion, it would be inefficient to use a muscle that flexes and side bends because that would be wasted effort. An example of this is the quadriceps or thigh muscles. When there is swelling on the knee, the inner one of the four thigh muscle may become less able to generate a force. The other three quadricep muscles may need to compensate by working harder to make up for the slacking inner quadricep muscle. However, the line of action of the force of the three remaining quadricep muscles is inefficiently angled slightly to the side.

The combination of the increased force needed by the three quadricep muscles and the angled line of action sets up the cartilage of the knee joint for overloading which may lead to damage and inflammation. Thus, one injury causing swelling of the knee may lead to compensations and tissue injury, and the compensation – overload – pain – compensation – cycle continues.

Are you someone who likes to "work through the pain" or goes by the philosophy of "no pain, no gain"? Perhaps, you are highly motivated to play in the game or landscape your yard or dance until the band stops playing. However, when your brain senses or anticipates pain, to protect itself, it may go into fear/pain-avoidance mode and use compensatory muscles to carry out the task. What "working through pain" may mean is that *compensatory* muscles are being challenged and strengthened. In the quadriceps example described above, this may mean strengthening compensatory muscles *and* overloading knee joint cartilage. It's best to use the right tool, that is the right muscle, for the right job. Have you ever tried to use manicure scissors that you have been using for years to open cardboard boxes? Frequent compensations may overload tissues leading to injury or an inability to function well when you need them for the job that they were meant to do.

CHAPTER 17

Movement Requires All of You: Physical, Emotional, Cognitive, and Spiritual

"Getting to know you. Getting to know all about you."
– Rodgers and Hammerstein[26]

What have you learned so far?

You learned about the parts of the movement system and how their shape and size determine their roles (Chapter 10). You know that pain is the body's method for communicating information to protect the body (Chapter 13). You know about fear/pain-avoidance movements, and that the body compensates to get the job done safely while minimizing pain (Chapter 16). What you need to know next is how your nervous system coordinates all your body parts to perform safe, efficient, and pain-free movement.

The trial-and-error approach that you may have been using to meet your movement goals may not be effective for you, which is why you are reading this book. *Know* first. *Do* second. Learn about how the nervous system works to create movement to help you make wise movement decisions (serotonin jolt for you).

The nervous system includes A) sensors that provide information about body parts to the brain, B) nerves that send information into and out of the brain, and C) the brain.

A. There are many sensors in the body. The ones that are important in movement include those that detect pain, touch, pressure, vibration, stretch, positions of joints, speed of movement, and head movements (vestibular sensors in the inner ear). Vision and hearing also are important sensors because they provide information about the surroundings.

B. Nerves are like the electrical wires in a car that transmit signals from sensors in the fuel tank, tires, and radiator to the dashboard which may be viewed by the driver. In the body, nerves carry information from sensors to the brain, to different parts within the brain, and from the brain to muscles.

C. The brain combines information from sensors located throughout the body, the surroundings, memories from previous movements, level of alertness, emotional state, and movement goals to develop a movement plan. This plan contains information on how much each joint should move, which muscles to use when and with what force, and when the muscles should rest. While movement is occurring, the brain is continually updated with sensory data which may be used to adjust the signals to muscles to perform the desired movement.

The Brain and Movement

The brain functions like a computer detecting and analyzing sensory information, communicating information to appropriate parts, and recalling previous experiences to meet future goals. Computers are made of hardware (computer chips, power supplies, cooling fans, etc.) and software (directions and guidelines). These work together to manipulate data to create documents, edit photos, pay bills, and more. The computer user inputs data by entering words, numbers, photos, or scanned documents, then manipulates the data using software programs in the computer, and finally outputs the new data to a printer or another computer or stores it for future use.

Like a computer, the brain receives data, manipulates it, and creates an output of movement. The information input to the brain may be categorized into five areas: physical and cognitive components, emotional state, spiritual intent, and the environment. All these components contribute to the performance of safe, efficient, and pain-free movement. It is important to keep in mind that movement involves the whole person, not just the visible physical parts. People may function in similar ways to a computer, but we are more than robots and our motivation to move plays a big role in movement.

As you already have read, the **physical components of movement** include all the sensors, muscles, tendons, ligaments, bones, special parts like cartilage and bursae, and nerves. The nervous system coordinates all these physical components to create safe, efficient, coordinated, balanced, and accurate movements.

Emotional state refers to level of arousal (alert or asleep or somewhere in between) and a corresponding level of activation of the sympathetic versus parasympathetic nervous systems (see Chapter 2). When there is chronic pain, there may be increased sensitivity (lower tolerance) to pain which may lead to early activation of the sympathetic nervous system. Once in the 'fight or flight' mode, there may be a higher tolerance for pain which means that pain may not be sensed until it is at a high level (hopefully before an injury occurs). In the sympathetic mode, muscles are prepared to develop force quickly. In contrast, in the 'rest and digest' or parasympathetic mode, muscles are more relaxed and easier to stretch. This is why stretching is more effective when combined with deep breathing. Both these modes of the nervous system may affect movement. Emotional state may vary from heightened awareness, to anxiety, to relaxed, to depressed. These moods may impact physical readiness to move and attention to monitoring the quality of movement. Level of motivation may also affect quality of movement. On a Friday before a holiday weekend, you may be thinking about how to arrange your patio furniture rather than how to move groceries from your car to your pantry using good body mechanics.

The **cognitive component of movement** is muscle or movement memory. Muscle memory is information the brain has stored from past movement experiences such as when to contract or rest a muscle, how much force to use, and how slowly or quickly a muscle should activate. Movement memory is a group of muscle memories that combine to accomplish a movement goal. Movement memory is developed by monitoring a movement for quality, accuracy, pain, speed, and refining the movement through repetition. In the early stages of learning how to move, movements are simple, performed slowly and are closely monitored for quality. With repetition, less monitoring is required since the muscles have memory of how to perform the task successfully and the movement becomes automatic or habitual and efficient. When there is movement memory, the brain may be able to attend to other tasks. For example, if holding a handrail to get into your residence is automatic because you have done it a thousand times, your brain may give more attention to what you need to do to get dinner ready. Or, if you are able to sit down safely and efficiently because you have done it thousands of times, you may be able to give more attention to finding just the right seat on the bus or subway when you are on your way to a job interview.

Movement memory and the ability to perform accurate movements efficiently are foundations for more complex movements such as climbing on wet rocks to get into a good position to take a photo of a lighthouse. Higher-skilled activities may require being able to adapt or revise an ongoing movement. A basketball player, who has the movement memory of bouncing a basketball while running, can focus on the defenders and adapt or revise his/her movements and decide when to pass the ball or take a shot. These skills make him/her a more valuable basketball player.

The highest level of movement is creating new movements, such as a new dance step or how to get dressed when your shoulder is in a sling.

With any movement activity, from playing the piano to constructing a bookshelf, building on simple movements that are performed well is a recipe for success. In movement, "Good practice makes good performance." Good practice means many repetitions of high-quality movement. Doing 20 volleyball serves at the end of practice with only five staying in-bounds is not good practice and does not provide good movement memory for good performance in a game. Hammering nails to the right depth each time creates good movement memory for the next nail. Being able to perform movements well without close attention because you have good quality movement memory frees up your brain for other important tasks. You may focus on figuring out how many more boards you need to finish your project so you can get to the home improvement store before it closes.

The quality of movement memory improves with repetitions and deteriorates if it is not kept up to date. If there are changes in flexibility and strength, the old movement memories becomes less useful. For example, a person may have good movement memory of getting up off the floor at age 50. However, at age 70 if their speed of muscle contraction is slower and their knees don't bend as well, movement memory from 20 years ago may not be helpful. Ideally, the person would have continued to perform getting up off the floor over the years to have movement memory that pertains to a 70-year-old body.

'Weekend warriors' may get injured because they do not keep up with their flexibility, strength, or movement memory, or they engage in movement challenges beyond their abilities. The movement memory of being an outstanding ice skater as a teenager may have negative consequences for a 30-year-old who tries to show off their spins to their friends at the annual holiday skating party. Think safe, efficient, and pain-free movement and get a neurohormone jolt for making a wise movement decision.

The **spiritual intent** of movement is a person's purpose or goal for doing a movement. When shoveling snow for a neighbor, is the intention to have a good physical workout, make money, have a reputation as the fastest snow-shoveler on the block, or make a big pile of snow so you can have fun building an igloo? The amount of physical, emotional, and cognitive effort dedicated to shoveling and how the snow is shoveled (quickly, sloppily, precisely) may be different depending on the intent and the goal.

The component of the **environment** impacts the safety of movement. The levelness, texture, and friction of the support surface, the amount of light, the weather, physical obstacles, and time constraints are all environmental factors that are accounted for by the brain when developing a movement plan. A person's clothing, footwear, braces, and sport equipment are environmental factors that may limit some motions, resulting in movement compensations. If the environment is changing while the movement is progressing, there may be a need to make modifications to the movement plan. For example, if you slip on wet grass, your very next step may be shorter or you may walk slower to help prevent a fall. Your 'genius car' in action!

CHAPTER 18

Maximizing Your Movement Options

The combination of all the components of movement – physical, emotion, cognitive, spiritual intent, and the environment – generates many potential options to accomplish a movement goal. The number of options vary with the person, their age, emotional state, movement experiences, goal, and the environment. You may increase your options by improving the functioning of the physical, emotional, cognitive, and spiritual components (Table 5).

Table 5: Movement Components

Component of Movement	Role of Component	Possible Actions
Physical components: muscles, bones, ligaments, bursae, sensors, etc.	Flexibility, joint range of motion, strength, endurance, sensing vision, hearing, touch	Stretch, strengthen, challenge speed of movement and endurance, release scar tissue
Emotional component	Prepares body emotionally for movement	Increase alertness or decrease anxiety, replace negative emotional states with positive ones
Cognitive component: movement memory	To improve efficiency of movement	Increase repetitions of good quality movements
Spiritual component: goal	Provides motivation	Make clear goals with time frames
Environment: lighting, weather, support surface, physical obstacles, time, footwear, clothing, braces, equipment	To maximize safety	Improve lighting, remove obstacles, reduce time constraints, select footwear, clothing, and equipment appropriate for the movement

Returning to the car analogy, options for movement are like the roads on a road map. You may choose from many roads to get from Seattle to Galveston. The number of options will be less if you are driving a semi-trailer that can only be driven on highways, and more if you are on a motorcycle that can travel on any type of road. With movement, if you have poor balance and are limited to walking on even surfaces, you have fewer options than someone who has the physical abilities to take the shortcut up the grassy hill.

There are many paths on the brain's road map for getting from Point A to Point B. Each path is unique based on current information of the physical components, emotional state, movement memory, goals, and the environment. It is easy to drive a car on a wide, paved road that is well-lit which is like a person who has many components of movement to meet their movement goals. It is more difficult to drive a car on a narrow, gravel road without lights which is like a person who has fewer components of movement. If it starts to rain or the driver needs to get to their destination faster, the driver on the wide road is in a safer situation than the driver on the gravel road. With movement, having more options because you have more components increases the likelihood of being able to meet your goals safely.

Road construction may require the driver of a car to choose another path. In the body, pain, injury, or a change in the emotional state or goal may block your 'road' and require your brain to choose another path to accomplish a movement. For example: you want to finish a race, but your hamstring is having a painful spasm. To overcome your hamstring problem, you have choices. You could change your emotional state by putting up with more pain than you usually do and anticipate your friends congratulating you on your good time, or you may change your goal of having a fast time, slow down, and congratulate yourself on taking care of your body. Life may be more pleasant when you have more options for movement, which means having more of each of the five components available as shown in Table 5. In movement rehabilitation and in healthcare in general, it is important to communicate goals clearly. Then providers may suggest interventions to improve your components needed to reach your goals.

When physical components of movement are lost due to injury, pain, age, or other reasons, easy movements may become difficult (Chapter 8, Figure 1). You may be aware that you are losing options for movement. Many patients say, "If I don't do something now, by the time I am 65, I won't be able to attend my nephews' and nieces' weddings, go bird-watching, or volunteer at the annual fundraiser."

Try getting up from a chair after a knee replacement or meniscus surgery. Typically, the quadriceps would be called upon to get into standing but that option might not be available because of weakness of the knee muscles due to pain and/or swelling. Try playing table tennis when you have foot pain. Not being able to use your foot to get into position quickly may result in a shoulder injury from overreaching. Some other ways that you may lose physical components of movement are wearing unsupportive footwear or poor-fitting clothing, muscle fatigue, wearing a brace or sports gear like a helmet or gloves, having cold hands and feet resulting in decreased sensation, obstructed vision, and poor hearing. All the above detract from the sensory information that is necessary for good movement. Or you may have been diagnosed with neuropathy which is decreased or altered sensation typically of fingers and toes. You may compensate for a loss in sensation by tightening your finger or your toe muscles, but that may decrease the coordination needed to place a cup of coffee on a glass table or balance while walking.

What Are <u>Your</u> Options for Movement?

If someone recommends that you use a cane, instead of rejecting the suggestion because "I don't want to feel old," you may consider saying, "Thank you for increasing my options for movement. I know that since I have lost some sensation in my feet, I have lost some options for movement, and I am at a greater risk for falling. The cane gives my brain extra information about the location of my body and more options to restore a loss of balance." A restaurant server may set a goal for their movement program of "I want to improve my options for movement by improving my agility and the reaction time of my feet so I can work faster and make more money." It is good (as well as safe and efficient) to have a lot of options when you need a new plan for movement due to changes in muscle function due to fatigue, an unexpected change in the environment or your emotional state, or if the movement goal changes.

Be proactive. You are a 30-year-old who sits at a computer most of the day. You tell your co-workers, "I am going to support my arms on the desk when I use my keyboard and mouse and let my shoulder muscles relax. I know that I have the option of using either my shoulder muscles or the desk to support my arms. When I use the desk, I have no shoulder tightness at the end of the day, and I can play hockey after work without worrying about having pain or tightness in my shoulders."

For successful movement, like a computer, 'garbage in equals garbage out.' Poor quality data in terms of the physical components – flexibility, strength, muscle endurance, sensory information – has greater potential for 'garbage out' or movements that are unsafe, inefficient, and painful. When you make a cake, you probably make sure you have all the correct ingredients and that they are fresh. You are not substituting powdered eggs for real eggs, and your baking powder is not 20 years old. When you build a picnic table, you use boards that are not warped and screws that are not rusty. In movement, when you are lifting, you don't want to overload small back muscles because you have not kept up with strengthening your quadriceps. If you are changing an inner tube on your bike, you set up the surroundings with good lighting, so you don't injure yourself with the wrench when you replace the tire on the rim. With movement, you may have your cake (or be able to make another cake) and eat it too (be happy about meeting your movement goal) if you replace the ingredients that you used up by stretching muscles that became tight with activity, rehabilitating muscles or joints that were injured, or replacing worn out shoes.

In life, people who are successful sometimes overcame a tragedy in their early years and spent a lot of effort trying to avoid another one. When no tragedy materialized, they ended up being successful and happy because they were able to distance themselves from potentially negative situations. They valued themselves and prepared before acting. They 'looked before they leaped.' Avoiding negative consequences was their reward. The same strategy may be applied to the movement system. Improving physical components of movement and increasing movement memory is rewarded by not having to sit on the sidelines when others are continuing to play, work, travel, and enjoy physical activity.

Here are some tips to help 'keep your motor running.' A more extensive list is presented in Chapter 21.

1. Maintain the function of the physical components of movement: muscle flexibility, strength, endurance, and speed of muscle contraction, joint range of motion, and senses such as vision, hearing, vestibular, proprioception, and tactile (Chapter 30).

2. Use good posture and movements throughout the day to train fundamentals of movement (Chapter 25) and enhance movement memory.

3. Know how body parts are supposed to be used and how they may be injured (Chapter 10).

Let's do a quick review, and then we'll go on to some examples of making wise movement decisions.

What Have You Learned?

You *know* that you are the owner of an awesome movement system. You know that you have an amazing brain that makes decisions quickly for you as you move safely and efficiently throughout your day. And you know that you have a communication system that signals pain when movement needs to be adapted or stopped to maintain safety and efficiency.

What you need to *do* is improve your understanding of how your body parts work, use the parts correctly, and listen to the signals your body is sending you, particularly pain.

Movement Scenarios

Persons A, **B** and **C** need to replace an overhead lightbulb in the middle of a room.

Thirty-year-old **Person A** has never changed a lightbulb in their house because they just moved in. They are in good physical condition. Although they have no applicable movement memory of replacing a light bulb, they have a lot of well-functioning components for movement (sensation, flexibility, strength, speed of movement, joint range of motion.). And they have a chair, a step stool, and a ladder and a 2-year-old child who wants to play.

Person B is 70 years old, and their spouse was the last one who changed the lightbulb 10 years ago. They have some limitations in shoulder range of motion and vision. They have no movement memory of changing a lightbulb and fewer available components compared to Person A. They have a chair and a step stool but not a ladder. Because of their deficits in components of movement, no applicable movement memory, and not having a ladder, they have limited options to accomplish the movement.

Person C works in building management and has been changing at least five overhead lightbulbs a week for the past 20 years using a chair, step stool, and ladder. They are a bit overweight and are less flexible than Person A, but they have a lot of movement memory, which increases their options for movement.

Person A changing the lightbulb should make sure that the environment is safe and not rush the movement because their toddler wants to play.

Person B may want to try to increase the range of motion of their shoulder and practice reaching overhead using the step stool near a wall to increase their movement memory before they try to change the lightbulb in the middle of the room. To be safe, they need to plan the movement carefully and closely monitor the progress.

Person C might consider stretching before they change the lightbulb to minimize their need to compensate for restricted joint ranges of motion.

In another example, a football coach has a team which includes linebackers, running backs, wide receivers, and a quarterback each with different physical components and movement memories based on their position. The coach also knows that the turf is slippery at the 20-yard line, how much time it takes to run plays, which players work better under pressure and which plays have been most effective in the past in scoring touchdowns. The coach has gathered data on the physical, emotional, cognitive, and spiritual, and environmental components to make wise decisions on which players and plays have the greatest potential to score a touchdown (meet the movement goal). The coach assesses the outcome of each play and if things are not going well, they may choose to get off one road (set of players and plays) and turn onto another one on their road map. To meet the goal of winning the game, the players may benefit by focusing their training on skills that are specific to their position. A wide receiver may practice changing directions quickly and a lineman may work on staying upright when a 300-pound person tries to knock them over. Both players may want to perform their movements on wet turf and grass, so they have some movement memory if it starts to rain when they are playing in a game.

Another movement scenario is a person who awakens from sleep with the thought, "I have to go the bathroom." They know they need to plan their movement because last time they were in this situation they almost fell. They wisely think, "I am going to do move my legs around before I get up because my muscles and joints are stiff from lying in bed for four hours (physical component). I remember that there is a raised threshold (environmental obstacle) between the bedroom and the bathroom, so I will make sure I pick up my feet when I get there like I learned in physical therapy (movement memory and calm emotional state). I have some hip stiffness that limits my options, so I need to take short steps." Suddenly, the person realizes they need to get to the bathroom quickly or they are going to have an accident (environmental constraint of need for speed). The person compliments themselves because they prepared for getting up in the middle of the night to go to the bathroom by putting their walker next to the bed and turning on the night light. To improve their options for movement, the person may choose to 'put money in their ability bank' by practicing walking quickly in daylight then advancing to nighttime lighting since their need for speed often occurs at night.

These examples show that movement scenarios have a wide range of physical, emotional, cognitive, spiritual, and environmental components. Being aware of all of them and attending to them as needed increases options for movement and the likelihood for experiencing safe, efficient, and pain-free movements.

CHAPTER 19

Putting It All Together or "What's Going on Under the Hood"

When making a presentation, the process is to tell people what you are going to tell them, tell them, and then tell them what you told them. Repetition is necessary for learning – sounds a lot like muscle and movement memory and 'good practice makes good performance.' With practice, even difficult and complex movements may be accomplished without much thought, that is, focused attention. Your 'genius car' in action!

You may need to focus on how you are moving when you are having pain or you are trying to improve a movement. The following concepts of movement may help you, your healthcare providers, and your movement instructors solve your problem. This list was created from over thirty years of being a physical therapist. Some of the concepts may be familiar to you from earlier chapters and others will be presented in later chapters.

1. The main priorities of movements are that they are safe, efficient, and pain-free. For survival, the brain selects movement plans that minimize injury to body parts or the experience of pain. Efficient use of resources means using body parts in the way they were meant to be used based on their shape, size, and tissue type (Chapter 10). Efficiency also means conserving the body's energy by limiting the use of extra body parts to perform a movement. This may be done for example by wearing sneakers to help keep the foot and ankle stable when walking on uneven surfaces rather than wearing unsupportive footwear like open-back sandals, flip-flops, or clogs.

2. The performance of a movement relies on a) up-to-date accurate sensory input, b) the physical, emotional, cognitive, spiritual, and environmental components of movement, c) a movement plan or option that accounts for the five components of movement, and d) the ability to adapt or modify the movement if there are changes in the physical and cognitive components, emotional state, goal, or the environment.

3. Sensation is very important in movement. You can't get there from here if you don't know where here is. In other words, you need to know where you are starting from to be able to get to where you are going. If you want to go to New Hampshire, the direction you go in will be different if you start in Montana or Arkansas. Incomplete sensory information and pain may interfere with safe and efficient movement. Remember the dot-to-dot game you played as a child where you connect the numbered dots to outline a shape? If there is a large distance between dots, or you skip some numbered dots, you may not be able to figure out if the shape is a giraffe or a vase. In the body, more dots is the same as more sensory information to the brain. If the brain does not sense the toes on the floor (as in neuropathy), it may not know if the toes are available for the movement plan. It may be challenging to stand on one foot or turn quickly to avoid walking into someone in a crowded store if you don't use your toes.

4. Deficits in sensory data may lead to muscles tightening up or going into spasm. When the brain 'loses' the location of a body part because of lack of data, it may compensate by a strong muscle contraction in that area, which gives the brain information on the location of the body part. Carpenters who frequently hit their thumbs with a hammer or someone who opens child-proof containers repeatedly may experience a loss in sensitivity to touch. Thumb muscles may go into spasm because of a decrease in sensitivity of the thumb due to repetitive trauma. In another scenario, when the ground is slippery, there may be a tendency is to take small steps and tighten up leg muscles to compensate for decreased sensation of the foot on the ground. The brain may create sensory information, tighten a muscle for example, to improve the safety of the movement.

5. A loss of sensory information due to an injury may persist long after a body part has healed. The injury may be gone but not forgotten by the brain. Chapter 14 explained

the body's inflammatory/anti-inflammatory/remodeling response to injury. The body puts a 'bandage' – scar tissue – on the injury to protect it as it heals. With bigger injuries, there may be more potential for scar tissue. Can you feel when someone touches your skin that is covered by several bandages (a lot of scar tissue)? If the brain is not getting useful sensory information from a body part, it may assume that the part is not available for use in the movement plan, and it may select another part to perform the movement (see the dot-to-dot discussion in #3 above). The memory of an injury may remain long after the injury has healed. You may have injured your leg when you were a child that is impacting your balance now. The brain stores information about movement continuously. Retrieval is another matter. As a 40-year-old, you may share with your teenager how you made the winning soccer goal when you were a sophomore in high school with two defenders in front of you on a windy Friday night because you were motivated to store the memory. On the other hand, some people do not remember which ankle they sprained or even that they sprained an ankle. Fortunately, healthcare providers with special training may be able to detect an old ankle injury by observing your movements and by doing a hands-on assessment.

6. The scar tissue formed in the healing process following an injury may cause body parts to perform at lower than pre-injury levels because of restrictions in tissue mobility and/or decreased sensation. These restrictions may result in decreased flexibility and 'strength' and/or decreased joint range of motion. This in turn may lead to overloading of other body parts to compensate for the lost function of the injured part.

7. Tissue injuries that undergo the healing process with potential for scar formation include muscle strains, ligament sprains, bruises to muscles or bones, or fractures which is the same as breaking a bone. Surgical cuts and abrasions may also result in scar tissue as well as diagnoses ending with -itis (bursitis, tendinitis, arthritis).

8. Tissue overload may be due to using a body part too early in the movement, too late, for too long duration, too quickly, or with too much force. For example, while foot pronation is a normal movement, *early and sustained* foot pronation may lead to excessive flattening of the arch of the foot. This may result in overloading of

the big toe which may cause toe pain. Another example is late contraction of the abdominals or poor core stability, which may cause an overuse of back muscles when lifting. Muscles may get injured during weightlifting when a muscle suddenly gives out to protect itself and the remaining muscles may develop large forces quickly to prevent dropping the weight. The brain errors on the side of safety and may produce a muscle contraction stronger than necessary when it doesn't know what to expect. The brain is doing its best to satisfy your goal of not dropping the weight, if your goal is to look strong in front of your friends (oxytocin jolt).

9. Pain is the body's communication system that relays information like a traffic light. Red refers to acute pain, which means stop the activity because an injury has already happened. Amber represents chronic or 'compensatory pain,' which means slow down, assess the situation, be prepared to stop the activity, and proceed with caution. Green is for 'good pain' which means keep going. 'Good pain' might be useful to help diagnose the *cause* of movement problems.

10. Pain is a symptom and may not be the problem. An old hand or wrist injury may be causing compensatory movements at the shoulder causing shoulder pain. When one sacroiliac joint (the pair of joints that connects the triangular bone below the spine to the pelvis [Figure 3]) is not moving well, sometimes it is the opposite one that speaks up in pain because it is moving too much and is causing irritation and pain. In both these examples, lasting improvement is more likely if treatment is directed at the *cause* of the symptoms – the part that is not functioning well – and not the one that is complaining of pain. In a work environment, it is the person *not* doing their job that is the problem not the person who is working frantically and making mistakes because they are doing the work of two people.

11. When a body part is first injured, the body goes into survival mode. Pain and swelling may inhibit muscle function and, to meet the movement goal, other muscles and joints may be activated because of the anticipation of pain. The movement is called a fear/pain-avoidance movement, which may lead to a cycle of compensation – overload – pain – compensation.

12. 'Functional weakness' may be due to pain, swelling, muscle fibers not sliding well, too much resistance, or trigger points in a muscle. Any of these may inhibit a

muscle from developing a force. Here is an example of 'functional weakness.' You wake up in the middle of the night because your child or grandchild is crying in the next room. A month ago, you bruised your thigh muscle on the corner of the desk. Your thigh muscle may be 'weak' from pain, swelling, and scar tissue. You are half asleep. Your thigh muscles have a big challenge, because of all the above inhibitions, to get to your child or grandchild quickly. There is a good chance you may experience a buttock or back spasm to compensate for thigh muscle 'functional weakness.'

13. Movement happens quickly, so you may not be able to consciously use an injured part if the brain decides to not use the part to protect it from further injury. 'Walking off' an injury may mean taking a few steps to figure out how to compensate and still be able to move at a functional speed.

14. Movement is planned in the brain using information obtained from previous movements (movement memory). The warm-up period before a game gives players the opportunity to recall movement memory by practicing free-throws, jumping, or making quick turns. It is important to warm-up before any activity where speed or endurance is required to provide the brain with current information on the environment and the physical components of movement (sensation including pain, flexibility, strength, etc.).

15. The body's ability to compensate is extensive but there may be a limit. A movement that was performed yesterday may not be possible today. "I just reached over to get something out of a box and my back went out." That last straw was the one that broke the camel's back. You may be unaware how close you are to injury because you are compensating well, or perhaps you have been ignoring the warning lights on your dashboard (the signals from your body).

16. The movement system is highly redundant. This means that the body has many muscles and joints and therefore a lot of possible combinations that may be used to accomplish a movement such as picking up a shoe from the floor. (See the example of teams A, B, C in Chapter 16.) There are five components that may affect the number of available options: physical abilities, emotional state, amount of movement memory, the goal or intent, and the environment. For instance, walking up wet stairs carrying packages in both hands wearing high-heeled shoes and the

train is about to leave the station presents a challenge to the brain to perform the movement safely. Aging, injury, and fatigue may decrease available options and may lead to overstressing the parts that are still contributing to movement.

17. Maintaining stability of one part of the body is necessary for mobility at another part. Core stability is a prerequisite for limb movement, which is why many movement programs incorporate core stability or abdominal strengthening.

18. Standing balance is achieved by the brain integrating information from vision, the vestibular system, proprioceptive, and tactile sensors. Having the eyes closed while performing an activity puts a greater reliance on the functioning of the latter three senses to maintain balance.

19. Movement memory is established in the brain when movements are performed repeatedly. When there is movement memory, less monitoring is required for performance and the movement is more automatic.

20. Muscles may become less flexible and shorten when they are not mobilized on a regular basis. When a muscle is stretched several things happen. Stretching aligns the fibers in a muscle, improves the ability of muscle fibers to slide on each other, and increases circulation to improve the removal of waste products from muscle contractions. When the brain receives an appropriate signal ('this muscle needs to be longer'), typically by stretching, it causes more muscle units called sarcomeres to form which makes the muscle longer. Flexibility, the ability to function as a longer muscle, may improve because restrictions to gliding of fibers are overcome **and** the muscle is physically longer. Frequent stretching reminds the brain to keep the additional sarcomeres to maintain the needed length of a muscle. Someone who sits most of the time without stretching may have shortened hamstring muscles. The message the brain receives is that the hamstrings don't need so many sarcomeres so some of them may be resorbed (taken away) so the body does not waste resources by keeping them available for use.

21. When challenged, muscle strength may improve by two processes: hypertrophy and neural adaptation. With excessive loading as when lifting heavy weights, the brain receives a message to increase the number of myofibrils which are the building blocks

of a muscle fiber. This increases the size of a muscle (called hypertrophy), which results in increased strength. Improving strength also occurs by a second process called neural adaptation. The neural pathways that are used for recruiting muscles become more efficient and coordinated and muscle memory is gained. For example, a couch may be moved more efficiently when there is coordinated effort, which means everyone lifts at the same time and walks in the same direction together.

22. To make a change in the body as well as in life, it is important to clearly state the goals. If you don't want your child to eat cookies before dinner, you may softly request. "Please don't eat the cookies before dinner." However, you may be more successful if you sternly state, "No, you may not have cookies before dinner!" With strength training, if your goal is to be able to carry a gallon of water (8 pounds) from the refrigerator to the dining-room table, lifting one pound 50 times is going to be less effective or perhaps not effective at all compared to gradually building up to lifting an 8-pound weight and then lifting it repetitively.

23. The number of blood vessels in muscles increases with aerobic exercise (movement that causes increased heart rate and increased amount of oxygen to tissues). Having more vessels means more oxygen to muscles, which improves endurance and delays the onset of muscle fatigue.

24. The body has processes for preventing muscle fatigue (explained in the next section) and for telling you when a muscle is fatigued. Using the car analogy, a warning light on the dashboard may tell you that your car is reaching its limit of function – there is only a small amount of fuel left. In the body, one warning light for muscle fatigue is trembling. Muscles may shake when they are not able to safely develop the desired force any longer. This might be a sign that a muscle is about to stop functioning and another one will need to compensate. If you keep trying to make a fatigued muscle contract, it may become overloaded and injured. Hopefully, your brain will have recruited a compensatory muscle before the fatigued muscle is injured or the movement needed to be stopped abruptly. However, now you are in the compensation cycle which may be leading you down a road that you don't want to be on.

Connecting the Brain to the Muscle – The Motor Unit

A motor unit consists of a nerve cell and all the muscle fibers that it innervates (sends a signal to). The motor unit receives a message from the brain via a nerve and the nerve cell sends a message to muscle fibers to contract or generate a force. What follows is a simplified explanation of how motor units generate a muscle force.

1. The number of motor units in a muscle varies between muscles. The number of muscles fibers that are attached to a nerve cell also is different depending on whether a muscle is used for fine control or for strength. In muscles that are used for dexterity, like finger and toe muscles, the nerve cell controls fewer fibers for more precise control of movement. This is in comparison to muscles that function more for strength like the thigh or buttock muscles where one nerve cell controls many fibers in order to generate large forces.

2. When a motor unit is activated, all the fibers attached to the nerve cell contract together and develop a force.

3. During a muscle contraction, the nervous system coordinates which motor units in the muscle are active and which are resting.

4. Muscle fibers use energy to contract and develop a force and energy runs out after a while (like a car that runs out of gas and stops working). The amount of time that fibers can maintain a contraction varies depending on the type of fibers in the muscle. The fibers that can contract for longer times are called Type I and the ones that have less endurance are called Type II. (There are also other types, but we'll keep it simple here.) Type I fibers tend to be slower to contract and have more endurance like the lower calf muscles, while Type II fibers tend to contract quicker but have less endurance like the biceps. Muscles may have a combination of Type I and Type II fibers, but usually one type predominates based on how the muscle is used during movement.

5. The amount of force that a muscle needs to develop to meet a movement goal determines how many motor units are activated at one time: in general, more motor units with more muscle fibers for a large force, less motor units with fewer fibers for a small force.

6. The 'genius' part of the force generation is this: the nervous system automatically switches between active and resting motor units to keep the total muscle force appropriate for the task. It knows when to let some units rest and replenish their resources and when they are ready to generate a force. When all is well, going between active and resting states is smooth and the desired muscle force is maintained. You don't notice the motor units switching on and off.

7. Muscle fatigue may occur during exercise or movement which in general refers to a muscle that is less able to produce a force. When muscles fatigue, they may start to tremble because there are not enough muscle fibers contracting well to maintain the desired force. You may feel that the muscle is becoming less strong. If you chose to keep doing the movement, there are some possible options: a) keep trying and overload the muscle which may potentially cause injury, b) stop and let the muscle rest to regain its ability to generate a force, or c) keep doing the movement and let the brain choose how to compensate with another muscle.

8. When part of a muscle is injured or inhibited, there may be less force from the muscle fibers of that motor unit. This may lead to a shorter rest period for other motor units which may cause a muscle to fatigue sooner.

9. Why can you hold a two-pound weight with your arm out to the side for several minutes, but your muscles start to tremble after a short time when holding a ten-pound weight? Muscle fatigue might be the answer. For the safety of your muscles, it might be a good idea to 'listen' to a 'muscle trembling signal' that might mean "your muscle is fatigued."

The take-home message: when you are engaged in a strengthening program and a muscle becomes fatigued, you may be strengthening a compensatory muscle. While doing a movement, it may be difficult to know when you are compensating. Patients have said to me, "I had no idea that I wasn't using the right muscle. Now I see that I can only do three repetitions when I use the right muscle." If your goal is to improve strength, you may consider seeking guidance from someone who is experienced in identifying compensations to assist you in learning the postures and movements that are safe and efficient for your body and your movement history.

CHAPTER 20

Misconceptions About the Movement System

Sometimes no knowledge is better than wrong knowledge. The following is a list of misconceptions about the movement system that I hear from patients.

1. **Incorrect:** 'No pain. No gain.' This implies that if you are not having pain, you are not gaining muscle strength or endurance. What you may be doing if you continue to exercise while having pain is putting yourself at risk for injury. (Note that some types of strength training may cause minor, painful tissue overloading that heals and results in increased strength. I recommend professional guidance if you are training at that level.)

   Correct: Some pain may be ok such as stretching, deep massage (controlled pain) or delayed onset muscle soreness due to eccentric muscle training. However, pain that is due to overloading body parts that results in significant inflammation is not ok because it may result in scar tissue, which may lead to a loss of function.

2. **Incorrect**: If there is no pain, there is no problem. 'No pain' may mean that your brain was smart enough to compensate. That is probably not a road you want to travel on for a long time.

   Correct: You may have no pain, but you may have a problem. The problem is that you may be compensating.

3. **Incorrect:** Because tissue has 'healed' and is pain-free, it is now flexible and strong like it was before it was injured.

Correct: 'Healed' tissue may no longer be painful, but depending on the amount of scar tissue that was formed in the healing process, the 'healed' tissue may not be as flexible or as strong as the tissue was before it was injured.

4. **Incorrect:** After an injury and the pain is gone, and the injured parts have been stretched and strengthened, they will automatically be used again in movements.

   Correct: Because of fear/pain-avoidance movements (Chapter 16), you may be compensating and using other muscles to perform your movements. Palpation of both the muscle to be trained and the potentially compensating muscles provides information on the timing and quality of muscle contractions and the onset of fatigue, all important for the return to safe, efficient, pain-free activity.

CHAPTER 21

Preventative Maintenance for Your Body

Here are some tips to help keep your movement 'car', your body, on the road:

1. Past medical history: Keep track of all major and minor injuries and medical conditions that may have affected your ability to move. The Appendices provide diagrams and charts to fill out and keep updated. This information in the hands of healthcare providers and movement instructors may help to identify the cause of compensatory pain. A knee sprain at age 7 may still benefit from treatment at age 90. Fill out the forms for yourself and your children. Your movement team will be grateful (oxytocin jolt).

2. Learn about the parts of your body and how they work together to produce safe, efficient, pain-free movement. (Chapter 10 on body parts and Chapter 19 on concepts of movement.) Use body parts in the way they were meant to function.

3. Take care of your feet – the eyes of walking. Foot care includes the skin, circulation, swelling, sensory changes such as numbness, tingling, or burning, joint mobility, muscle flexibility, muscle strength, wearing footwear that is protective, supportive, and has good traction, and addressing pain that is persistent or that interferes with balance or walking.

4. Have regular checkups of eyes and ears. Vision and hearing give you early alerts about the environment that the brain may use to select safe, efficient, and pain-free movement options. Reduced acuity (having blurry vision) or vision field loss (parts of what is in front or to the side is absent) may interfere with balance. Hearing a dog barking a half block away allows time to prepare to

modify movements if necessary. This is safer than having to attend to an uneven sidewalk and being startled by a barking dog at the same time.

5. Keep hydrated based on the recommendations of your healthcare provider. Muscles need water so the fibers may slide over each other to elongate (stretch) or shorten (contract to generate a force). Dehydrated muscles tend to spasm more readily than hydrated muscles. Lower than normal levels of blood circulating in the body, due to dehydration, may cause dizziness when moving from sitting to standing quickly which may cause a loss of balance or a fall.

6. Promote overall health with good nutrition and sleep. Engage the 'rest and digest' parasympathetic nervous system to promote healing. Realize that the 'fight or flight' nervous sympathetic system engages with stress of all forms – even anxious thoughts may stimulate the sympathetic system. Increase the release of 'feel-good,' happy neurohormones by doing behaviors that are rewarding (dopamine), promote feelings of connectedness or social well-being (oxytocin), and increases the respect from others or pride in yourself (serotonin). Monitor emotional health. Make goals that use movement to get 'feel-good' neurohormone jolts **and** the benefits of physical activity.

7. From my experience, I recommend a thorough evaluation of your movement system every year or two starting at age 50 or earlier if you had physical injuries as a child, to identify compensatory movement patterns before they present as pain. Consider a hands-on assessment to identify tissue restrictions due to 'old but not forgotten by your brain' injuries that may inhibit muscle function and lead to compensations. Restrictions in tissue that interfere with muscle contractions typically do not show up on imaging tests but may be sensed by touch. The goal is to restore any losses of physical function to increase options for movement. The 'bandages' or scars from old injuries may still be with you even though you don't feel them (Chapter 14).

8. Preventative maintenance for your physical body may include stretching, strengthening, and cardiovascular and muscle endurance training.

9. Prepare for new physical activities gradually and with guidance if you are unsure how to proceed.

10. Wear protective clothes and shoes that are appropriate for the activity. Use the correct tools and equipment sized to fit you (exercise equipment, computer desks, etc.).

11. Carefully consider participation in childhood sports that may be too challenging for the child's physical abilities such as wearing cleats before the feet and ankles are strong enough to manage the instability, or engaging in contact activities with other children who are much larger, stronger, or faster.

12. Be aware that physical and cognitive fatigue (see #13) may increase your risk for injury.

13. Distractions may reduce the ability to monitor a movement for safety, efficiency, and fatigue. Examples of distractions include noise, a busy environment, or trying to solve a problem that requires cognitive attention.

14. Pain is your communication system – your yield sign, red light, or flashing red light at a railroad crossing. Listen to the message. Stop and assess. It may be in your best interest to rest, modify, or stop the activity.

15. Consider professional guidance to recover from injury or to improve performance rather than trial-and-error and shot-gun approaches. Learn about your strengths and weaknesses and set appropriate goals.

16. Become familiar with the risk factors for falling for yourself and others. There are many questionnaires that help to identify fall risk.[27-28] Some of the risk factors include: a medical history that includes a loss in a physical component of movement like a stroke or Parkinson's disease, blood pressure that lowers upon standing, taking several medications or medications to help with sleep or mood disorders, visual and cognitive deficits, foot pain or decreased sensation, the need to rush to the bathroom quickly, use of an assistive device like a cane or a walker or holding furniture while walking, needing to use hands to get up from a chair, history of a fall, and a fear of falling. If you feel you are at risk, have an evaluation to identify your specific issues.

CHAPTER 22

Fine Wines Age Well: Tips on Being a Fine Wine, *Not* a Fine Whiner

The circle of life. We are born with little movement ability, we practice and learn routine and skilled movements, then we gradually lose some of the components that are needed for safe, efficient, pain-free movement. Ideally, along the way we gain movement memory and wisdom to make wise movement decisions. Changes that may occur with increasing age that cause movement to become slower and more deliberate include[12,29]:

1. Diminished sense of touch at the feet may impact balance.[30]

2. Loss of vestibular sensors in the inner ear. When you move your head, the vestibular system is activated to help you maintain your balance. If this response is too slow, you may lose your balance when you turn quickly to check how the pot is doing on the stove (Chapter 30).

3. Vision and hearing losses decrease the accuracy and the quantity of environmental cues needed for safe movement.

4. Decreased sensation of thirst and less fluid intake[31] or there may be purposefully less drinking of fluids to avoid having to go to the bathroom frequently. Insufficient amount of water in the body may lead to dehydration, muscle spasms, and lower blood pressure.

5. Decreased sense of taste may lead to decreased appetite with potential for nutritional deficits.

6. Loss of muscle mass and strength called sarcopenia.

7. A reduction in the size of fast-twitch muscle fibers that are used for quick movement. Known as Type II fibers, these muscles fibers are used for high-intensity bursts of activity, such as rapid movements to get across the street quickly before the light changes or reaching to catch something before it falls.

8. Postural changes due to decreases in sensation, joint range of motion, strength, and endurance.

9. Slowing of the transmission of information through the nervous system. There may be a mismatch between movement memory and the physical components necessary to carry out a movement.

10. Slowing of the brain's ability to change from one task to another.

Aging and Movement Components

With all the losses of **physical components** listed above, in normal aging, movement typically becomes slower. Less sensation of the toes means more time and more weight may be needed for the toes to sense the floor before a movement may occur or proceed.

Question: What is the difference between a young person walking on ice and an older person walking on a dry, level sidewalk who has lost some physical components of movement?

Answer: There may not much be of a difference!

Both the younger and older person move slowly and carefully and may tense up a lot of muscles doing so. And both may have sensation concerns. The younger person walking on ice may feel that their feet might slide out from under them at any time. The older person may have diminished sensation of their feet, so it takes longer for them to feel the ground. Prolonged 'walking on ice' may lead to muscle fatigue and stiffness because the gait is slow and deliberate to help prevent a fall. The older person may benefit from a cane to increase the sensory information of body location which may allow for quicker movements with less muscle guarding and muscle fatigue.

As people get older, a fear of falling, anxiety, or depression may cause a negative **emotional state** that may impact movement and the motivation to move.

With increasing age, the **cognitive component** of movement memory may be less due to a more sedentary lifestyle, or movement memory may not apply to current physical abilities.

With increasing age, there may be physical limitations that make it more challenging to **set goals** to get 'feel-good' neurohormone releases. How do you get social needs met (oxytocin) if you can't play golf and have lunch with the guys or climb up a bleacher to watch a baseball game? Or how do you feel if you are not able to prepare Thanksgiving dinner anymore (serotonin)? Is it possible to anticipate a travel experience (dopamine) if you don't know how well you will be able to walk in a month?

Rather than sitting around and complaining about what isn't, a lifetime of adapting hopefully has provided you with wisdom to make the best of a situation.

"God, grant me the serenity to accept the things I cannot change, courage to change the things I can, and wisdom to know the difference." Reinhold Niebuhr (1932-1933)[32]

This quote may be applied to movement. To paraphrase, acquire the serenity **(emotional maturity)** to accept the things **(physical abilities)** you cannot change, courage **(spiritual)** to change the things you can, and wisdom **(cognitive knowledge about movement)** to know the difference.

Tips on Being a Fine Wine

Get medical clearance and seek professional guidance before starting new activities that involve your movement system.

1. Learn how your body parts are meant to be used.
2. Add to sensory awareness of the feet by massaging and exposing the feet to different surface textures (safely).
3. Improve muscle strength (neural adaptation and muscle hypertrophy (Chapter 19) by regular physical activity and by increasing the resistance or difficulty of your exercise and/or movement programs.
4. Practice rapid movements to stimulate Type II fast-twitch muscle fibers and to

create movement memories that are applicable to daily activities.

5. Repeat a task varying the speed, lighting, background distractions, level of fatigue, and the environment (height of stairs, furniture) to increase movement memory and the ability to adapt to movement challenges.

6. Perform movements of the whole body to improve balance and coordination for functional activities like reaching, lunging, and getting up off the floor.

7. Practice changing from task to task and performing novel tasks to stimulate the brain.

8. Consider the intervention of visualization/motor imagery.[12-13,20] Performing artists, athletes, public speakers, and people in rehabilitation use visualization to 'practice' the movements they are going to do when they are 'on stage.'

CHAPTER 23

Documenting Movement History

When you visit your healthcare provider, your medical record is updated so that your provider can identify trends in your health, responses to medication and other interventions, and to monitor current health issues. If you change providers or go to a specialist, your health history is usually readily available via electronic medical records.

From the perspective of a physical therapist, having a medical history of your physical body would be useful information when evaluating and treating your movement issues. What childhood injuries did you have? Were there any traumas like bike or car accidents or broken bones? Have you had any surgeries that may have created scar tissue that may be interfering with your muscle or joint functions? Sometimes people forget that they even had an injury or which leg was broken. Even if you don't remember having an injury, the tissue in your body does. Your brain also knows about the old injury because it may be having you perform compensatory movements to avoid using that body part. A hands-on assessment may help to identify tissue that was injured even decades ago. Manual assessment is done by sensing the subtle differences in tissue texture and the resistance to pressure compared to uninjured tissue. From my experience, typically there is tenderness at the site of an old injury.

The Appendices give you four charts to fill out to document the history of your physical body:

- ▶ Trauma, Surgery, Skeletal Asymmetries
- ▶ Pain, Weakness, and Other Symptoms
- ▶ Interventions to Improve Movement
- ▶ Lifetime Activity Level

The first three are necessary; the fourth is optional but providing all the information may help make the evaluation and treatment of movement issues more efficient.

I recommend filling out the forms for your children as injuries occur. Memory has a way of fading with time. It sometimes has taken several physical therapy sessions for people to recall an injury that happened long ago. The information on the physical health history forms may be used by your healthcare providers and movement instructors to create individualized exercise and movement programs to maximize your movement abilities and performance.

You are now ready to move on to the Doing part of the book. Congratulations on persevering through Part 2 and gaining a lot of knowledge about the movement system (serotonin jolt). I hope you will enjoy sharing what you have learned with your family, colleagues, patients, and clients (oxytocin jolt). Your reward for investing time and energy in Part 2 is a page away in Part 3. It is amazing that you transitioned from a baby, who had to be carried, to someone with a vast repertoire of skilled movements. Your 'genius car' in action!

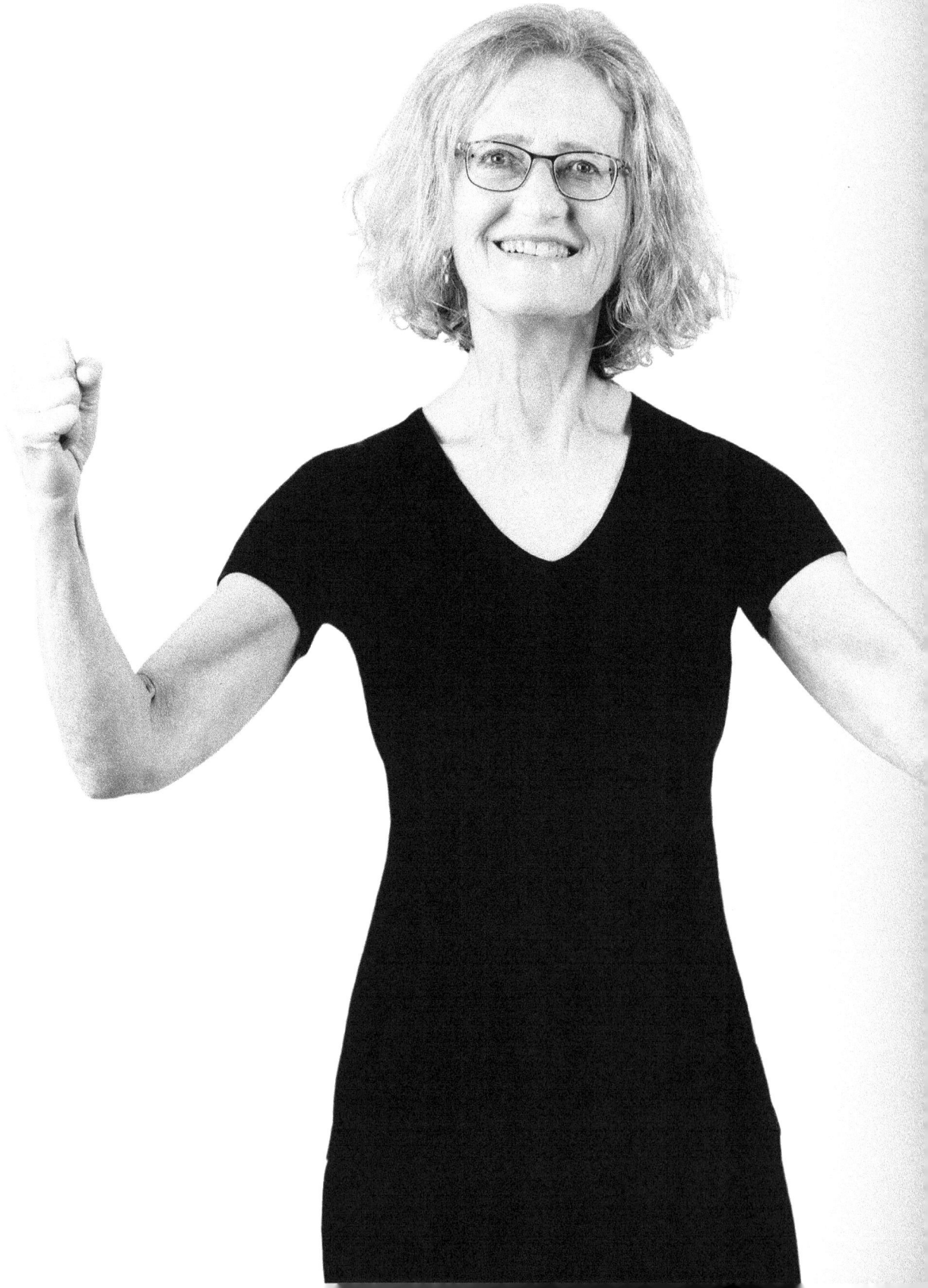

3
Doing

"The eye sees only what
the mind is prepared
to comprehend."

– Robertson Davies[33]

Applying Robertson Davies' quote to movement, 'After there is *comprehension* of movement, you are prepared to *see* movement.' In Part 2, you were provided with knowledge to be able to *comprehend* movement. Now, you have the opportunity to *see* movement.

Here is where the rubber hits the road – your 'car' in motion. In Part 3 **Doing**, you will have the opportunity to learn about:

    A. movement fundamentals

    B. how the environment may affect movement,

    C. movement memory,

    D. preparations for movement, and

    E. a process for observing postures and movements.

What Happens Next?

Chapter 24 presents how movement develops from a baby lying in a crib to someone who can get out of a bed, into and out of a car, play soccer, or assist Grandpa out of a chair. The goal is for you to be able to see when fundamentals of movement are being performed well and what it looks like when a fundamental is not being performed well.

Chapter 25 presents six fundamentals of movement which are based on my entry-level and post-graduate physical therapy education.[18,21,34] Other instructors of movement who work with patients or people who have specific work, recreational, or sports-related movement goals may use different strategies when they perform movement analysis. The fundamentals that will be used in Chapter 30 to analyze movement are:

    1. *good postural alignment, stability, and endurance*

    2. *good stability then good mobility*

    3. *maintaining balance by keeping the center of gravity within the base of support*

    4. *good support surface contacts*

5. *using support surface contacts to shift body weight while maintaining good postural alignment*

6. *weight acceptance while maintaining good postural alignment and balance.*

Once these fundamentals of movement can be performed well, movement progresses to more complex and faster, skilled movements. Higher levels of movement include adapting movement in a changing environment or with changing goals and creating new movements. This book focuses on 16 postures and movements that are typically performed on a weekly if not daily basis.

As an infant and toddler, you practiced and learned fundamentals of movement all by yourself without studying a book or watching videos. Starting from lying on your back playing with your hands and feet, to rolling over, crawling, and walking you progressed through what is called the developmental sequence of movement. As you tried more challenging positions, postures, and movements you continued to perform the fundamentals. The goal of movement analysis is to break down a movement to assess what may be interfering with good performance. This type of analysis helps to identify why you (or your clients or patients) may be having pain during or after a movement activity or performance is not meeting expectations.

Chapter 26 *presents how the environment may affect movement.*

Chapter 27 *explains the importance of 'movement memory' for efficient movement.*

Chapter 28 *goes into some advanced 'Get Ready's' both physically and cognitively to help keep your 'car' on the road for a long time. This is followed by tips on planning movements and how you might assess if your movement program is 'steering you in the right direction.'*

Chapter 29 *presents a process for analyzing movement: what to look and listen for, and what the mover might be feeling and thinking.*

Chapter 30 *presents photos showing good and 'less than ideal' techniques of 16 activities to help you develop your movement analysis skills. The photos are critiqued using the language of the fundamentals of movement.*

CHAPTER 24

How You Got From Here to There in Your 'Genius Car'

The Developmental Sequence and
The Development of Purposeful Movement

Let's talk about your development from an infant needing help to hold a bottle to someone who rides a bike, goes to work, or cares for an elderly parent. Knowing how your body learned skilled movement may help you figure out why you may be having difficulty performing safe, efficient, and pain-free movements.

The car – body analogy. A car starts out with a fixed number of functions and ends up with the same number of functions just older, less shiny, and less able to accelerate quickly compared to when it was new. Your 'car' evolved from an infant who mostly stayed still and looked cute into a person who can roll, crawl, stand up, walk, run, go bowling, and repair the plumbing under the kitchen sink. Now that's 'genius!'

To get from an infant to a mobile person, you went through the developmental sequence of movement. The developmental sequence is a series of body positions and movements that build on each other to transition a person from lying on their back to being able to walk. The sequence is: lie on the back or stomach, roll, support self on stomach with extended arms, sit with support, sit without support, transition to hands and knees (quadruped), crawl in quadruped, kneel, stand, and walk. Sometimes some steps are skipped or are accomplished in a different order. Some infants don't crawl in quadruped and some toddlers run before they walk. Usually, this early 'running' is uncontrolled, and the toddler needs to use furniture or the ground to stop their forward momentum. With aging, the process may go in reverse. If components of movement are lost, the quality of movement may deteriorate or become unsafe.

The development of purposeful movement starts from simple, large body movements and progresses to complex, small, refined movements. Initially, support surfaces are large (lying on your back) and they become smaller (standing on one foot) as the fundamentals are mastered. With continued improvement in abilities, movement may be challenged by advancing from stable surfaces like a wooden or tile floor, to less stable surfaces like plush carpeting or hiking trails, or moving surfaces, like a bike, moving sidewalk, or a balance board. The knowledge of how movement develops may be used to help to identify which parts of a movement may need to be improved to meet safe, efficient, pain-free movement goals. First the **knowing**, then the **doing**.

CHAPTER 25

Fundamentals of Movement

Learning to move follows a progression just like any other type of learning – simple to complex. When learning how to write, you learned letters, then how to combine letters to form words, then sentences, then paragraphs. Skilled movement starts from basic postures and movements. It then develops into more complex and skilled movements, and sometimes into newly-invented movements like some of those crazy dunks that basketball players do. The development of purposeful movement is orderly in that, ideally, there is competency at one level before advancing to the next level. Hence the expression 'learning to walk before you can run.'

1. Postural alignment, postural stability, postural endurance

Movement begins with good alignment of body parts. If you ever have driven a car before and after a front-end alignment you know the importance of alignment. When the air pressure of one of your front tires is low, the car may not respond well, the ride may not be smooth, and the overloading of some car parts may have some expensive consequences. Having poor alignment of your 'car' is probably not the best way to start a road trip, perform in a dance recital, or work a 10-hour day as a home health aide. With your body, having good postural alignment is a prerequisite to having good control of movement (a 'smooth ride').

Postural alignment refers to the relative positioning of body parts. Poor postural alignment in the spine means that the vertebrae are not lined up in their normal curvatures – cervical lordosis (backward curve), thoracic kyphosis (forward curve) and lumbar lordosis (backward curve) with the head balanced on top of the neck bones. Poor postural alignment also may refer to a joint that is being stressed because it is at the end of its range of motion such as hyperextending the wrist when pushing a heavy object. Prolonged poor postural alignment is more of a concern than having brief periods of poor alignment.

There are several reasons why you want to avoid poor postural alignment. Firstly, poor postural alignment may require extra muscles to be used to keep joints in place and not moving. An example of this is looking down at an electronic device that is in your lap which challenges the tissues on the back of your head and neck. This poor posture may cause headaches and upper shoulder discomfort. Secondly, poor postural alignment such as keeping a joint at end-range position may stress ligaments and other soft tissue. If tissues are lengthened permanently due to overload, they may lose their ability to stabilize a joint. The term '**end-range positioning**' is used to describe this postural malalignment. An example of this is hyperextending the knees while standing. Hyperextension may stretch the soft tissue behind the knee and which may lead to poor alignment of the knee joint (femur and tibia) and additional stress on knee joint cartilage. Thirdly, poor postural alignment of the thoracic and lumbar spines may lead to back pain, stiffness, and difficulties with breathing and balance.

After you have good postural alignment, you need **postural stability**. A stable posture is one that can be maintained when challenged, such as keeping both feet planted on the ground when catching a ball or keeping your trunk aligned when you reach to get something out of a bottom drawer. Postural stability usually requires the use of muscles. Once that is achieved **postural endurance** can be obtained. Postural endurance means having the ability to keep a posture in good alignment for the length of time needed to perform the movement.

Spinal postural stability and endurance are accomplished with the core abdominal muscles at the center of the body. The main core muscle is transversus abdominis. It wraps around the body at the lumbar spine like a girdle or weight belt. When the transversus abdominis contracts, it stabilizes the pelvis and lower spine. Typically, before there is movement of any extremity, there is activity of the transversus abdominis.

2. Stability then mobility

Lying on your back and moving your arms and legs challenges the core trunk muscles' abilities to keep the pelvis and lower spine stable. First the trunk is stabilized, then the arms and legs move. In another example, when swinging the right leg to kick a ball, the left leg has 'controlled stability' so the right leg can have good mobility. 'Controlled stability' used in this book can be defined as having some movement at a joint yet maintaining stability. 'Controlled stability' may be accomplished by the shape of a joint, ligaments, or muscles. When kicking a ball with the right foot, the left hip has some movement but maintains the stability needed to stand on one leg. That is, the left hip functions for controlled stability while the right hip functions for mobility. The demonstrates that one body part can be used for stability or mobility depending on the movement. 'Genius car' in action!

Since this fundamental of good **stability then mobility** is very important for safe, efficient, pain-free movement, I will provide another example. Visualize lifting a can of paint off the floor with one hand. If the muscles around the shoulder blade are not strong enough to stabilize the shoulder blade on the trunk, lifting the paint can may cause the shoulder blade to move away from the trunk. A compensation for poor ability to stabilize the shoulder blade on the trunk might be increased use of the muscles to stabilize the attachment of the upper arm to the shoulder blade, the shoulder joint (glenohumeral). But the shoulder joint is supposed to be mobile, not stable when lifting a paint can. It is difficult for a joint to be stable, not move, and be mobile, move, at the same time. Stability of the shoulder blade on the spine is needed before mobility of the shoulder joint to pick up a can of paint. Stability then mobility.

Some of the body's joints are meant more for mobility, some more for stability, and some perform both functions well (Chapter 10). Problems may occur when the movement demands on the joint don't match the structure of the joint. For instance, the activity of 'standing on the hands' that is done in gymnastics requires the shoulders to be stable to support the body's weight. But the shoulder joint (glenohumeral) is meant more for mobility, so there will need to be significant muscle development to stabilize the shoulder joint.

In walking, is the hip stable or mobile? It is both, depending on the phase of the walking cycle – the foot on the ground or the leg swinging forward. And the foot? At times it needs to be mobile to be able to adjust to an uneven surface, and at other times it needs to be stable to support the weight of the body. In movement, if all joints are mobile, the body may collapse, and if all joints are stable, there is no movement. So safe, efficient, and pain-free movement requires coordinating joints that may be continually changing their stability and mobility functions. And all this is happening without you micromanaging it. Your 'genius car' in action!

Movements performed when the body is stable are easier and safer than when the body is moving. Physical therapy for back pain incorporates the fundamentals listed above. If you have gone through core stabilization training, you may have performed ball passes between hands and feet while lying on your back then arm and leg lifting exercises when in quadruped (hands and knees or all-fours). Then you may have progressed to strengthening the core muscles in a standing activity such as squatting. After that you may have moved on and added more mobility by simulating lifting groceries from a cart and putting them in your vehicle. The development of movement progresses from stable surfaces with large areas of support like standing on two legs while brushing your teeth to unstable surfaces with small areas of support like reaching to pick an apple from a high branch while trying to avoid stepping on fallen apples.

3. Center of gravity within base of support

To maintain balance, the **center of gravity (of the body)** must be **within the base of support**. The center of gravity (COG) of the body is located approximately at the second sacral vertebra (the part of the spine that is below the lumbar spine). The base of support (BOS) is the outer limits of the body that is in contact with a surface. When standing, your BOS is from the front of your toes to the back of your heels to the outsides of both feet. Reaching out with your arm and touching a walker, a piece furniture, or a wall increases your BOS which makes you more stable and less likely to have your COG be outside your BOS which may result in a loss of balance.

When might your COG be outside of your BOS? You are standing on a step stool, and you are reaching over furniture to fix a curtain or paint molding on the ceiling. Or, you are putting on your pants while standing and you haven't completely shifted your weight onto your standing leg. Or you bend down to pick up a piece of paper that you dropped, and you lean too far forwards. To keep your COG within your BOS to help prevent a loss of balance, you can increase your BOS by placing your hands or other body parts on nearby surfaces.

A lower COG is more stable than a higher COG. Toddlers and elderly people sometimes walk with bent knees and hips which effectively lowers their COG making them more stable and less likely to fall. In football, running backs keep their COG low to make it more difficult for their opponents to bring them to the ground.

4. Support surface contact

Support surface contact (SSC) refers to the location and area of the body that is in contact with a support surface.[34] SSC may be expanded to include: 1) the body part that is in contact with the support surface (ground, furniture, handrail) and how much of the body part is in contact with a surface (a finger vs a hand), 2) the ability of the body to sense what it is touching, and 3) the friction between the body and the support surface. Larger areas of contact, more sensitivity to touch, and less or no slippage between surfaces is the best SSC. In a poor quality SSC there may be a) a small area of contact, b) diminished sensation that essentially makes the contact area smaller, c) pain that may make someone try to avoid contact with a surface, and d) slipping between surfaces which may make the support surface unreliable to push off from (wet, icy, sandy, dry skin, slippery clothing or soles of shoes).

Why might you be more likely to fall in high-heeled shoes versus sneakers or if you have pain in your big toe? Because your SSC is decreased. Remember fear/pain-avoidance? If you are avoiding using your big toe, it may not contact the ground in a timely way to contribute to safe and efficient movement. Decreased functioning of the toe may lead to compensations at the knee, hip, and spine. SSC gives your brain information on where you are which is critical for setting up a movement plan to accomplish your goal.

A car analogy is your GPS that needs information on where you are starting from so it can provide you with a 'plan' to get you to your destination. Having good SSC information is important for weight shifting and weight acceptance, the next two fundamentals.

5. Weight shifting

Weight shifting is exactly what it sounds like, moving weight. There are two ways to shift weight: push off a surface with your hands or feet or any other body part or move body parts. Either of these weight shifting strategies changes the location of your COG. Your COG shifts automatically when you move your leg to take a step or if you reach to grab a coffeepot. Note that after you pick up a coffee pot, that pot becomes part of your weight, and your COG shifts in the direction of the coffee pot. When you lift an object, to keep your COG within your BOS, you keep the object next to your body. A safe strategy for lifting would be to increase your BOS before you pick something up. When lunging (one of the 16 postures and movements that will be analyzed), you increase your BOS and shift weight onto your leading leg to get closer to the item you want to lift.

Good quality weight shifting contributes to making a movement more coordinated: the COG or weight of the body is shifted the right amount at the right time. An experienced driver turns the steering wheel the right amount, at the right time, with smooth, controlled deceleration and acceleration. An inexperienced driver might continually adjust the steering wheel, start the turn too early or too late, slow down too much going into the turn or accelerate too fast coming out of the turn. In movement terms, the experienced or skilled 'driver' (person) is safe, uses minimal effort, and there is minimal or no overloading of the steering or acceleration/braking systems of the 'car' (body). Skilled weight shifting improves safety and efficiency, and minimizes overloading body structures.

An example of unskilled weight shifting is using too much momentum to get up from a chair and losing balance forwards. Another example is shifting from two-legged to one-legged standing and flailing the arms because of inadequate control of the foot and ankle muscles to position and maintain the COG within the BOS.

What might be causing poor weight shifting? Fingers and toes that typically are responsible for weight shifting may not be effective because of decreased sensation, pain, weakness, range of motion limitations, or you may not be able to use them due to injury. Weight shifting may be more challenging when you are using your arms to hold something or when you are wearing ski boots or a leg brace. If there is a loss of sensation due to neuropathy, weight shifting may be performed by moving the head, spine, or hips (compensations) instead of the feet. The ability to weight shift might also be affected by range of motion limitations throughout the body. Also, fear/pain avoidance and the anticipation of pain may impact weight shifting. Compensations due to poor quality weight shifting may interfere with efficient movement even before the intended movement has begun.

6. Weight acceptance

The next fundamental of movement is **weight acceptance** or receiving and managing the new COG safely, efficiently, and with no or minimal pain. Do the body parts that might be accepting the weight have adequate flexibility, range of motion, strength, and good postural alignment, stability, and endurance, and can they respond in a timely way? Is there concern for potential injury? Might accepting weight cause pain? A body part may respond to these questions by 'saying' "No, I am not going to accept the weight that you are trying to shift onto me." If the intention is to continue with the movement, the solution might be to compensate.

Here are two examples of weight shifting and weight acceptance. You want to get a closer look at a label on a box that is at waist level but your knee muscles don't have enough endurance to keep you in a mini-squat position for more than a few seconds. Your knees are rejecting rather than accepting weight. So, what do you do? You may compensate by bending at your back with the potential for overloading your back muscles. People who have had an ankle sprain may not accept weight well on the outside of their foot and ankle. The foot may be slightly off to the outside or weight acceptance may be slow and deliberate and not at a functional speed. Fear/pain-avoidance movements when repeated may become movement memory. Even when pain is gone and strength is restored, movement memory persists. Walking with the foot off to the side and delayed weight acceptance may decrease speed of walking or running.

What else needs to be in place for weight acceptance? The parts accepting the weight need to be ready. The SSC (a foot for example) needs to be large enough to be able to distribute the weight to avoid tissue overload and to be able to maintain the COG within the BOS for good stability. Injuries may happen when the accepting parts are not prepared in terms of postural alignment, stability, endurance, or ability to control the weight. You may be able to accept the weight, but you may need some time to get into a position of postural stability first. When you learned to drive a vehicle, you were taught to "leave a way out" especially in heavy traffic. In movement, it's a good idea to leave some options open to accommodate for potentially new challenges. You may be risking injury if you are using all your physical components of movement to move a heavy box and you have an unexpected shift in your COG and/or your BOS when your foot slips on the floor.

Summarizing Movement Fundamentals

To review, movement builds on fundamentals of good postural alignment, stability, and endurance, and acquiring stability then mobility, keeping the COG within the BOS, having adequate and appropriate SSCs, weight shifting, and weight acceptance.

The following example uses the language of movement fundamentals to describe someone walking while wearing a walking boot. In the boot, the foot and ankle can only function for **stability**, so some other joint like the hip needs to compensate for the loss of foot and ankle **mobility**. Walking in a boot compromises the '**stability then mobility**' fundamental. When the foot strikes the ground, the hip normally would function for **stability** to **accept the weight** of the body. However, the hip may need to be **mobile** to adapt to an uneven ground because the foot in the boot can't perform the mobility function. To increase the **BOS** to improve balance, the person might place the foot more to the outside. However, the **SSC** between the boot and the ground may be decreased because the person may not be able to put the boot down flat when it is out to the side. With a wider BOS, the amount of **weight shifting** to position the **COG within**

the BOS of the foot is increased which takes more time and muscle endurance. With time, the hip may speak the language of pain because it is being overloaded. The person may choose to avoid hip pain by spending less time with the boot in contact with the ground, that is limping, which may lead to overloading the opposite hip.

The Developmental Sequence and Movement Fundamentals

To learn about movement fundamentals, observe infants and toddlers. For hours babies lie on their backs and play with their hands and feet and gain core stability. Infants rock in quadruped (all fours) and develop postural stability and endurance of their shoulders and hips. They use a large BOS to maintain balance by a) having their hands on the floor in front of them when they first sit, b) knees far apart when starting to crawl, and c) feet to the side in early standing and walking. Some infants 'bear crawl' on their hands and feet (a large BOS) before attempting walking. SSCs are large in early ring sitting (where the legs form a ring) and in early walking (holding onto furniture or 'furniture cruising'). Watch infants and toddlers weight shift. They use every finger, every toe, the top of the foot, the knees, the elbows, the shoulder, and sometimes their head to weight shift. Toddlers keep their COG low by keeping the hips and knees flexed when learning to balance in standing. Toddlers gain trunk control in kneeling before standing to take advantage of the increased SSC from the contact of the floor on their lower legs. To gain movement memory, toddlers do hundreds of repetitions when getting from sitting into quadruped or from squatting to standing by the couch – a lot more than three sets of ten.

As a toddler gains control of the basic movements of transitioning between support surfaces and walking, they become more adventurous. Higher level movement goals require more flexibility, strength, coordination, and precision. With practice, movement progress to skilled activities such as climbing a ladder or playing hockey. Movements that are skilled require less monitoring because of movement memory. In skilled movement, muscles provide the right amount of force at the right time, and they rest when they are not needed. This improves the fluidity and coordination of movement. Picture yourself decorating a cake or throwing darts for the first time. When you start a new movement, you are likely tense and the movement is slow and deliberate because you are using a lot of muscles to achieve good accuracy. This slow, controlled movement is accomplished by simultaneously contracting muscles that work in opposition to each other like wrist flexors and extensors. This is called co-contraction. With practice you learn to relax your wrist extensors when you are flexing your wrist and the movement is faster and more fluid. The 'walking on ice versus dry sidewalk' example demonstrates co-contraction. To help prevent slipping when walking on ice, the knees may be positioned in partial flexion which requires co-contraction of hamstrings and quadriceps. Injury and aging may increase the tendency for muscles to co-contract which may result in less fluidity and coordination of movement.

Now for the opposite end of the life cycle. What may happen to fundamentals of movement with aging? Postural alignment may not be as good due to flexibility and joint range of motion deficits. Stability may be diminished due to sedentary lifestyles, abdominal surgeries, or pregnancy. Keeping the COG within the BOS may be accomplished by increasing the BOS by using a cane or a walker, 'furniture cruising,' or holding onto a companion. SSCs may decrease because of foot pain, arthritis, or sensory losses. Weight shifting and acceptance may be slower because of aging (Chapter 22) leading to slowness in movement. On the brighter side, to maintain or improve movement, a good strategy is to figure out which fundamentals of movement are not being performed well and why, and then engage in exercise and movement programs that address the deficits.

Besides the differences in physical components in young and older people, movement may be affected by the situation or context. Infants and children have little or no time constraints or requirements to perform accurately and movements are mostly for play or for curiosity. Movements of an older person usually have time constraints, the need to be accurate without too much experimentation, and the movement usually has a well-defined purpose. We look at these constraints in the next chapter.

CHAPTER 26

Movement and the Environment

"I made all my shots at practice but was lousy in the game." I got all the practice questions correct but I only got a 'B' on the test." What happened? The environment became more complex, so the activities may have become more challenging. The gym was noisy, and you may have gotten nervous because you were fearful of not doing well. There is a reason why football teams practice 2-minute drills at the end of practice when they are tired, in a noisy stadium, and while it's raining. The environment may impact the complexity of movement. Let's see how environments vary from least to most challenging:

1. Closed environment where nothing in the environment is moving or constraining, restricting, or limiting movement: lunge, squat, reach in a large space.

2. Constrained environment that is not changing: lunge, squat or reach and touch the handle of a drawer or a cabinet that is fixed (a constraint) or move in a small bathroom (restricted).

3. Open, changing environment: shopping in a store with people that are moving, crossing a street when the light is about to change, walking upstairs with changing heights of stairs, reaching to pet a dog that is moving.

Movement may become more challenging when you are holding a toy, a cup of tea, a shovel, or a baby. Improving your ability to move safely with good balance in familiar and unfamiliar environments may require more than strengthening exercises. An exercise is an activity such as lunging with weights to improve muscle strength and endurance (number 1 above). Exercises are good in that they may help to maintain or improve your body's physical components and increase your options for movement.

If your goal pertains to specific movements and environments, a movement program that accounts for these variables might be more beneficial than a general exercise program.

On to environments 2 and 3. You may not be able to perform movements that you learned in a closed environment (number 1) when you are in a constrained or open environment (numbers 2 or 3). A simple movement like a lunge that is done in a gym (closed environment) becomes more complex and challenging when performed in a crowded kitchen (constrained environment) or on a tennis court (open environment). Making dinner with pets or children underfoot may have some undesirable outcomes unless you have addressed the components of movement that are needed in that environment (quick turns and stepping over toys while holding the mashed potatoes). On a tennis court there are time constraints on the lunging activity if you want to get to the ball in time to make a winning stroke. It is important to make movement goals specific to maximize the benefits of your exercise and movement programs.

Here is a scenario of someone choosing an exercise program that does not precisely address their movement goal. The person wants to be able to improve their balance, so they feel safer walking around their neighborhood. They decide to walk on a treadmill daily for 30 minutes, and they usually hold a rail for safety. A concern might be that since they feel a need to hold a rail, they may have sensation and/or strength deficits. While treadmill walking has many benefits (see Chapter 1), there may be other exercises and movements that more specifically address the *cause* of their balance problem. In the short term, the person may want to consider using a cane which adds sensory cues on body location and increases their BOS to improve balance. The treadmill is a fixed environment with minimal balance challenges. When the person goes to their dental appointment, they may be in an open environment and perhaps holding a tote bag. Specific movement programs may be developed to increase movement memory that is applicable to the environment where the person may be functioning.

The take-home message: To get more out of your exercise and movement programs, be specific when you develop your movement goals and know which components of movement you need to gain or improve to help you achieve them. The components may be muscle strength, speed of muscle contraction, sensation, or another aspect related to your movement goal. Muscle inhibition from pain or old injuries, joint ranges of motion limitations, etc. may benefit from additional interventions. After components of movement are addressed, movements programs such as yoga, Tai Chi, and dance may be beneficial to help train movement fundamentals. Varying the environment (closed, constrained, open and changing) provides opportunities to practice postural alignment, stability, and endurance, weight shifting, weight acceptance, and increase movement memory.

Congratulations! You now are at the next stage: analyzing movement (serotonin jolt). As we move forward, keep in mind the fundamentals of movement: postural alignment, stability, and endurance, stability then mobility, center of gravity within the base of support, support surface contact, weight shifting, and weight acceptance. These fundamentals are what you are going to be looking for when you observe movement.

CHAPTER 27

Movement: Past, Present, and Future

Past movements provided you with movement memory which is stored in your nervous system along with current information on the other components of movement (sensation, flexibility, strength, endurance, etc.). All these components are used to develop options for movement – the same as having many roads (options) on a map to get you from Point A to Point B. For the driver of a car, the roads that are used more frequently are more predictable and easier to travel whereas the less-traveled roads require more attention and may be more difficult to navigate safely. The same is true for your movements. Some are easy to perform because they are automatic and need less monitoring. It is like assembling a bookcase or grilling a hamburger. If you've done the task before, you know which tools to gather ahead of time, you know the sequence of the steps to get to your goal, and you know which parts of the task you need to monitor to get a good outcome. When you 'drive your car' and travel new routes, you learn other ways to get to your destination. If your goal is to cook meals seven days a week, you may want to master baked chicken, vegetable soup, and tacos as well. Now you have more options for getting dinner on the table as opposed to making hamburgers seven days a week. When you need to change roads due to road construction (no hamburgers in the freezer or you are having pain when you bend your knee) you can easily choose another road that you have been on before (baked chicken or walking down a ramp instead of using the steep stairs).

As with any learning opportunity, it is best to start movement when you are young and continue to add to your repertoire as life goes on. You teach your child to scramble eggs, so they know that when they are 16 years old, cooking is an option for getting a meal versus texting for a food delivery. After mastering eggs, you teach your child how to make something more complicated like meatballs with sauce. To be prepared for any movement challenge such as holding a baby while walking upstairs, crawling in an attic, or running a 10K, you want to have a lot of components of movement available. You obtain these by engaging in a variety of movements that improve flexibility, strength, endurance, and coordination. Perhaps this explains why some professional athletes take up dancing in the offseason: Dancing adds to more movement memory of balance so when they are in a game situation, they have more road maps to choose from to get away from a defender. If you encounter a new movement challenge such as "fallen rocks ahead" in the car analogy, your expanded road map (movement memory) may enable you to approach the movement opportunity with confidence rather than fear. As you recall from Chapter 21, fear of falling is a risk factor for falls. Increasing components of movement and performing novel movement activities are good strategies to help decrease the risk of falling.

Present movement is what you are doing now, today. A current trend to improve health is to engage in a walking program. Consistent walking may improve movement memory which may allow for attention to be focused on meeting other movement goals like sightseeing while on vacation or finding your seat in a theater. Walking on a sidewalk (safely) versus a treadmill may allow for more opportunities to vary foot placement, joint ranges of motion, speed of movement, step length, cadence and more. Balance may be challenged even more by stepping over or avoiding obstacles on a sidewalk or walking on uneven surfaces like grass or gravel. All these variations may improve physical components of movement as well as movement memory to enhance the movement road map. **Use present time to gather movement memories to increase options for current and future movements.**

Ok, you've got your **past** movement memory, your **present** movement abilities, and you have a **future** movement goal of safe, efficient, pain-free movement. Hopefully you've been taking care of all the preventative maintenance for your body. Now it's time for some last-minute Get Ready's.

CHAPTER 28

Get Ready! Planning Movement

You need to get to the airport to get to your vacation destination. Get Ready! There's a list of things you need to do before you leave. Think of how the *italicized* actions words in the next paragraph might apply to a new movement that you want to do or an existing one that you want to improve.

You *choose* your clothes and *prepare* your medications to take with you. You may *check* the zippers on your luggage. You have a *plan* for how you are going to get to your hotel. You *select* appropriate shoes for traveling. You *assemble* and *organize* the contents of your luggage. You *coordinate* with your driver and *explain* that you want to get to the airport two hours before departure time. You *identify* which documents you need to board the plane. You *monitor* alerts on your phone for potential changes in your flight times. You *proceed* to your departure gate. When in-route, you *look at* the estimated landing time in case you need to *change* your ground transportation. You *adjust* your sitting posture to avoid feeling stiff. You *manipulate* your tray table so that your water is nearby, and you *operate* the buttons to give you better lighting while you are reading. You *maintain* the safety of your electronic device by putting the cap on your water bottle. The person next to you is using your right armrest so you *adapt* by holding your device in your left hand. You keep in mind that traveling is part of your vacation, so you *relax* and enjoy talking with fellow travelers and perhaps *create* a new friendship. When you get to your hotel you *assess* how the traveling went and how you might *design* your next trip so you may have an even more pleasant travel experience.

What actions were used to get you to your destination? *Choose, prepare, check, plan, select, assemble, organize, coordinate, explain, identify, monitor, proceed, look at, change, adjust, manipulate, operate, maintain, adapt, relax, create, assess, and design.* All these action may be applied to movement. Just like movement memory makes performing a movement easier, repetition of a process creates a memory of how to perform a process. You may be able to easily perform the steps involved in getting to your vacation destination because you have done it many times. The process that I am presenting in this book is about observing and analyzing movement. Like any other process, it is orderly, and skipping steps usually takes more time because you may need to go back to the beginning and address the steps that you skipped.

If you have had a learning experience that was frustrating, try to recall if a step of the learning process was skipped or if you were not competent at one level before you moved on to the next one. Perhaps someone gave you a recipe, but they forgot to tell you about one ingredient, or how to prepare it. After decades, I realized that I was frustrated with chemistry because I did not understand the periodic table well.

People who teach movement – coaches, parents, siblings, teammates, healthcare providers, personal trainers, yoga, kick boxing, and dance instructors – usually follow a process. One such process is called Bloom's taxonomy of learning.[35-38]

There are three areas or domains of learning in Bloom's system of learning: the cognitive (what to *know*), the psychomotor/technical (how to *do*), and the affective (valuing what you do, which is motivation for knowing and doing).[35-38] Each of these areas of learning has many levels beginning with basic knowledge or skills and progressing to higher levels. By incorporating these three areas, cognitive, psychomotor, and affective when teaching movement, the student may be more engaged and rewards may come more consistently. Recall that one step in the process of change is 'give yourself frequent rewards.' What is good about using a systematic approach to teaching with well-defined learning objectives is that if you encounter an obstacle in the learning process, you may go back to the levels of learning to see if steps were skipped or if competency was lacking at one of the levels.

Tips for Planning Movement

You already prepared your brain with knowledge about movement in Part 2. Some additional physical and cognitive aspects of movement are presented next that may be used to plan safe, efficient, and pain-free movements.

Physical:

1. Prepare body parts:

    a. Get rid of swelling – it may inhibit muscle function.

    b. Stretch muscles and other soft tissue (skin, tendons, ligaments, etc.)

    c. Move joints: a goal of gentle range of motion is to lubricate the cartilage on joint surfaces and the cartilage between bones. Cartilage may be compared to a rubber gasket in a car. When a gasket is dried out or when cartilage is not lubricated well, it may have less ability to conform to irregular surfaces, and therefore it may be less effective at dampening forces when compressed.

    d. Know the limitations of the mover(s) so movements may be stopped when approaching a danger zone (a better strategy than having to stop after having gone too far).

2. Assemble and prepare the right equipment for the task: footwear, kneepads, exercise equipment sized appropriately with the right resistance, stepladder, or other necessary equipment.

3. Assess and prepare the environment and identify any potential hazards: floor is dry, area is not cluttered, and lighting is adequate.

4. Allow enough time for the movement.

5. Communicate with everyone involved in your movement. Discuss how you are going to do the task. Be in position to observe the other people that are involved in the movement to make sure they are not doing something that is unsafe or has the potential to be unsafe. If they have a problem, you may be the

one left holding the weight. Discuss not rushing the movement. Agree to stop the movement at any time. If you or the other person state they need to stop in the middle of the task, stop first and ask questions later.

Cognitive:

1. Monitor and respond to the body's warning signs – pain, overstretching, numbness, fatigue, or a feeling that something is not right.

2. Avoid keeping joints and muscles in their end-range position for prolonged times to prevent damage from overstretching muscles, tendons, ligaments, and other body tissue.

3. The ability of a muscle to generate a force may depend on the length of the muscle (shortened, midrange, or lengthened). This length-tension relationship may explain why as the elbow approaches full flexion and the biceps muscle is in a shortened length, your biceps curl may feel weaker.

4. After completing the movement, assess to help prepare for the next movement – what might be done the next time so the movement may be easier, safer, or you can have more fun doing it.

Are You on Track to Meeting Your Movement Goals?

Here are some indicators that you are moving in the right direction:

1. You are demonstrating improvement. You can get up from the couch in one attempt instead of three. You can run two miles without soreness.

2. You are having less pain.

3. The movement seems to flow easier. You don't have to pay as much attention to how you are moving.

4. You are not tired or achy afterwards.

5. You are adding more resistance or duration to the movement. You are doing the movement faster or with better coordination or accuracy.

6. You are trying more challenging movements that require more balance or coordination.

7. You readily engage in activity. You are looking for more ways to move versus looking for excuses not to move.

8. You are confident in trying new movements in new environments.

9. You are having fun!

CHAPTER 29

Get Set! Preparing Your Senses to Analyze Movement

Part of physical therapy education is one-on-one mentoring by experienced therapists in various clinical settings. In my first meeting with one clinical instructor I was asked "What do you want to learn?" Of the many topics that we needed to cover, she wanted to know my goals so she could prioritize my learning experience. I answered that I wanted to know what she saw when she observed a movement, how she used her hands to assess and treat movement, and how she used what she saw and felt to identify the deficits that interfered with the person's ability to move.

In addition to providing you with knowledge on how the movement system works, this book offers information on observing and analyzing movement.

Some people don't understand why they are still having pain after receiving and participating in physical therapy and other interventions, resting, exercising, changing the way they move, and/or buying expensive footwear. Maybe they were not successful because the interventions were not addressing the *cause* of the movement problem. Perhaps they needed to have their fundamentals of movement assessed: postural alignment, stability, and endurance, stability then mobility, center of gravity within the base of support, support surface contact, weight shifting, and weight acceptance.

We will start by observing and analyzing photos of movement that are part of the development sequence. Then we will look at postures and movements such as reaching and lunging that demonstrate good technique and poor, compensatory strategies. The goal is to use the combination of the *knowing* from Part 2 and the *doing*, observing movement, from Chapters 29 and 30 to help find the *cause* of pain and/or poor performance with movement.

Perhaps a two-year-old asks "why" at least 20 times a day because they want to know how things work so they can control their world better. Patients ask me "why" because they are tired of being in pain and tired of spending time and money on interventions that don't improve their symptoms or performance. Like any root-cause-analysis, the process is to repeatedly ask "why" to focus in on possible *causes* of the problem. Compliance officers, managers, and 2-year-olds choose a root-cause-analysis strategy to solve a problem because it is more methodical and directed compared to trial-and-error or shotgun approaches.

Get medical clearance and seek professional guidance as necessary if you are considering performing any of the positions, postures, and movements shown in the photos. There may be limitations of your posture, joint range of motion, or muscle usage due to a surgery, injury, disease process, or other reason. If someone is directing your movements, like a coach, trainer, or therapist, make sure to inform them of any of these limitations or any adverse responses you had to movement in the past.

You may be thinking that you can observe your movements by looking in a mirror. Realize that by changing your head position to look at yourself in a mirror, you are not getting a true picture of your posture or weight shift. Some movement instructors take videos of their clients to help them see their movement deficits. Also, movement changes with repetition so it is a good idea to view several trials of a movement. Athletes compensate very quickly. If they perform a movement that demonstrates poor balance on the first trial, by the second trial they may have already compensated and are showing you 'good' balance.

The following postures and transitional movements used in everyday life demonstrate fundamentals of movement presented in Chapter 25. The photos show when the fundamentals are present and when they are lacking.

1. Lying on the back reaching hands to feet

2. Rolling from back to side-lying

3. Reaching while lying on the stomach

4. Sitting on the floor

5. Transitioning from lying on the stomach into quadruped (hands and knees)

6. Transitioning from sitting on the floor into quadruped

7. Transitioning from sitting on the floor to standing a) via quadruped with furniture, b) via quadruped without furniture

8. Sitting in a chair – posture

9. Moving to the front of a chair – weight shifting

10. Transitioning from sitting in a chair to standing a) with hands, b) without hands

11. Mini-squatting and hip hinging

12. Picking up shoes from the floor

13. Standing on two legs

14. Standing on one leg – balance

15. Lunging forward – reaching

16. Lunging to the side – reaching

Information on movement comes from seeing, hearing, and input from the mover.

Here is what to **look** for in the photos:

1. Posture: Is the alignment between body parts good? Are any joints in an end-range position? Is there left to right symmetry? Are body parts being used for their intended function? Does it look like some part is compensating? Does it appear there is too much effort being used to maintain the posture? Is there control of the postures or does it look like collapse or loss of balance may occur if the posture or movement is continued?

2. Is the core (pelvis/lumbar spine) stable. Do the joints bearing weight appear to be stable?

3. Is the center of gravity (COG) within the base of support (BOS)? As the positions progress through the developmental sequence from lying to standing, the BOS will become smaller and the COG higher. Both require more postural stability and endurance. While a large BOS improves stability when crawling in quadruped or walking, it also requires greater weight shifting which may interfere with forward progression.

4. Is there good support surface contact (SSC)? Is the area of contact between the surface and the body appropriate for the activity – such as the foot on the floor, the thigh/buttock on the chair? As development progresses from lying to standing, SSC decreases which requires more postural stability and endurance.

5. What part of the body is causing the shifting of body weight – fingers, toes, movement of body parts (head, arms, legs), body leaning? Is postural alignment maintained during the weight shifting? Are compensations used to maintain balance?

6. What part of the body is accepting the weight? Is there good SSC using the correct body part and is it adequate for the weight it is about to accept? Is postural alignment maintained and controlled or are there compensations to maintain balance? Has the body part accepted weight? Does it seem like some body parts are straining to maintain balance?

Here is what the mover might **feel** as they do the posture or movement:

1. Is there pain, numbness, pins and needles or any other sensation that is unusual?

2. Is there a sense of the whole foot, hand, or other body part on the surface when appropriate, or does it feel like some of it is not in contact with the surface?

3. Are there any muscle sensations: stretching, straining?

4. Does anything feel stiff?

5. Is there a feeling that a muscle is about to give way, spasm, or fatigue?

6. Is there a delay in a muscle's activity?

7. Do any muscles feel like they are working too hard or too long?

8. Does it feel like one joint or muscle is doing all the work?

9. Does it feel like some muscles are not doing anything when it seems like they should be working?

10. Does the posture or movement feel stable?

11. Does the movement feel coordinated?

Here is what the mover or observer might **hear** when the posture or movement is taking place:

1. Are joints crackling or clunking?

2. Is the foot slapping on the ground or is there a pounding sound as if a body part may be accepting weight too quickly?

Here is what the mover might be **thinking** as they do the posture or movement:

1. Does the posture or movement require too much work to sustain?

2. Does the mover want to stop because it seems like something not good may happen?

3. Does something not feel right?

A deficit that is subtle might become more obvious when the posture or movement is performed with the eyes closed. When taking away visual information, there is increased reliance on sensation to maintain balance. *(Safety precautions such as having someone nearby should be in place when movements are being performed and especially when a movement is being performed with the eyes closed.)* There may be a greater chance for loss of balance when a movement is performed with the eyes closed. A posture that appears and feels balanced with eyes open may look and feel different when the eyes are closed. Ask the **look, feel, and think** questions again and there may be different answers.

Even more information about fundamentals of movement may be gained from a movement analysis if compensations are not allowed. Examples of compensations might be knee hyperextension or movements of the arms to help maintain balance. Eliminate compensations and ask the look, feel, and think questions again.

To summarize, the skilled movements that you are doing now are based on fundamentals of movement that you learned when you were an infant and a toddler. Higher level skilled movements like sports and hobbies also rely on movement fundamentals. These more complex movements usually happen quickly so they may be more challenging to observe and analyze. A good way to start learning about observing and analyzing movement is to become familiar with where to look to find deficits in movement fundamentals.

CHAPTER 30

Go! Analyzing Movement

The first four postures and movements show how infants gain fundamentals of movement abilities in about six months usually with no formal instruction. 'Genius car!' Take your time and read these sections sequentially, view the photos, and become familiar with the terminology. Once you become comfortable with the language, you may be better able to focus your attention on analyzing the photos to be able to see if fundamentals of movement are present or absent.

1 | Lying on the back reaching hands to feet

The hands reaching to the feet while lying on the back is the beginning of core muscle strengthening (Figure 33). Moving the arms and legs away from the trunk challenges the core muscles to stabilize the spine. When there is good core stability, the spine remains flat on the surface (or slightly lordotic) (Figure 34). If core strength is inadequate, the back arches excessively (Figure 35). A progression to improve core strength and endurance is to add weights to the hands or feet.

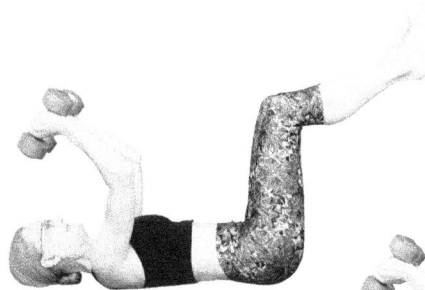

Figure 34

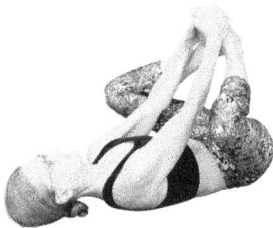

Figure 33

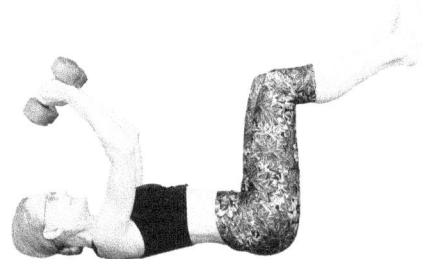

Figure 35

2 | Rolling from back to side-lying

Good core strength is necessary to maintain spinal postural stability during rolling from the back to the side as when getting out of a bed (Figure 36). A good technique to assist 'log rolling' and limit rotation of the spine is to push off the surface with the back foot (Figure 37). A poorer strategy for getting out of a bed is demonstrated in Figure 38. As the person rolls from their back to their left side, they use excessive back and neck extension and thrusting the pelvis forward to shift the center of gravity (COG) onto the left hip. Figure 39 shows another poor strategy for getting out of a bed – rocking forwards until there is enough momentum to shift the COG of the body onto the right hip. The problem with using momentum to shift the COG is that if the weight shifts too far forwards, there may be a loss of balance if the COG moves outside the base of support (BOS). To stop the forward momentum and help prevent a loss of balance, some other part of the body needs to react quickly to stop the movement. Obviously, using momentum to change body positions may be a risky strategy.

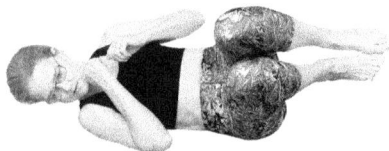

Figure 36

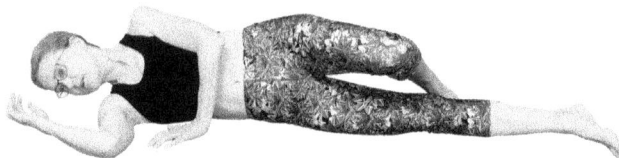

Figure 37

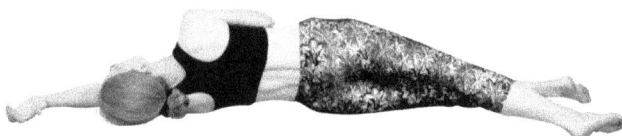

Figure 38

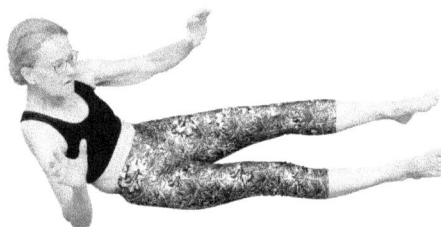

Figure 39

3 | Reaching while lying on the stomach

The activity of lying on the stomach and reaching demonstrates all six fundamentals of movement: 1) Good postural alignment, stability, and endurance, 2) Stability then mobility, 3) COG within the BOS, 4) Good support surface contact (SSC), 5) Weight shifting, and 6) Weight acceptance. Development progresses from lying on the stomach with the arms at the sides to propping on forearms (Figure 40), to reaching while propping on forearms (Figure 41), to propping on hands (Figure 42), and to reaching while propping on hands (Figure 43). Fundamentals of movement that are demonstrated in the prone prop position:

1. The spine is in good alignment throughout the movement with good postural stability and endurance.

2. There is stability at the shoulder blades otherwise the shoulders might be elevated compared to the trunk or the trunk might be lower and closer to the surface.

3. The COG of the body is within the BOS.

4. There is a large SSC of the trunk and forearms on the floor.

5. Weight shifting is accomplished by pushing from the right forearm and hand which shifts the COG of the body to the left. With the body weight off the right shoulder, the right arm is free to reach forward.

6. The left shoulder and forearm accepted the weight well as the left shoulder remains in good alignment with the trunk. If the weight is not accepted well, the trunk may lower to the surface.

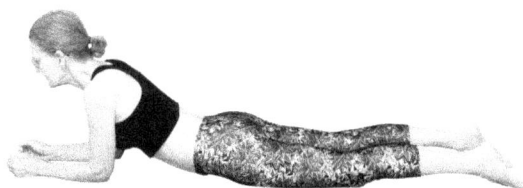
Figure 40

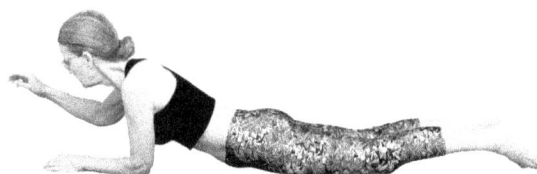
Figure 41

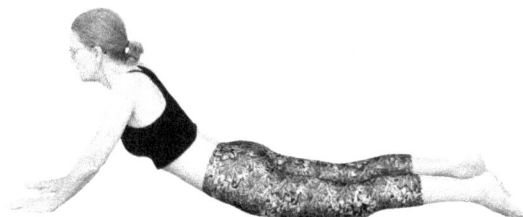
Figure 42

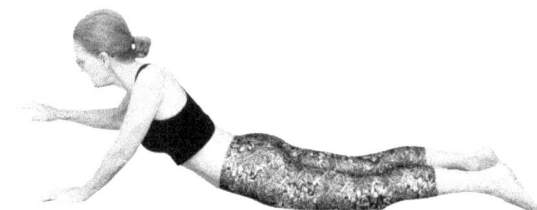
Figure 43

4 | Sitting on the floor

Usually, infants are first placed in sitting and supported by a cushion of some sort and later they learn how to get into sitting by themselves. An infant may sit without a cushion by using their hands for support and a wide BOS of the legs (ring sitting) (Figure 43). Since the back muscles are not strong enough to hold up the trunk, the hands, and feet may be used to shift the COG back onto the buttocks to help prevent the trunk from falling forwards.

Figure 44 ring sitting shows poor spine postural alignment, poor postural stability of the trunk, the COG within the BOS, and a large SSC of the buttocks, lower legs, feet, and hands.

Figure 45 cross-legged sitting with hands on thighs shows a progression in development as the BOS from front to back is decreased compared to Figure 44. Postural stability of the trunk is lacking as demonstrated by a flexed trunk.

Figure 46 cross-legged sitting with hands on thighs shows a more erect trunk demonstrating an improvement in spinal postural endurance compared to Figure 45.

Figure 47 cross-legged sitting with hands free to play demonstrates further improvement in spinal postural stability and endurance, which allows the infant to have mobility of the arms. Reaching forwards and to the sides improves core stability, weight shifting, and weight acceptance onto different parts of the legs and thighs in preparation for transition into quadruped.

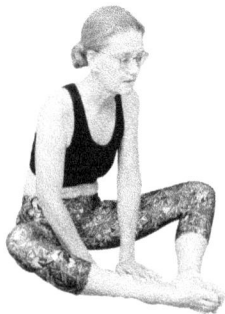 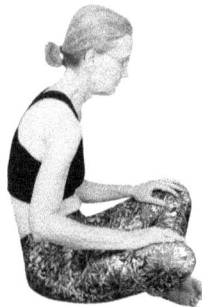 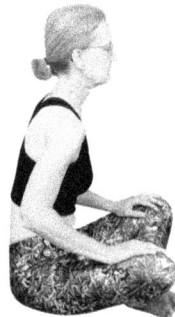 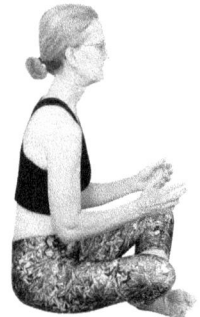

Figure 44   **Figure 45**   **Figure 46**   **Figure 47**

5 | Transitioning from lying on the stomach into quadruped (hands and knees)

Figures 48-52 show two ways to transition from lying on the stomach to quadruped. The first strategy (Figures 48 and 49) uses the arms to shift the COG towards the legs in one motion. Then the hands are 'walked' backwards, or the knees are 'walked' forwards until the hands are in line with the shoulders and the knees are in line with the hips (Figure 50). This strategy uses minimal side to side weight shifting, which suggests a lack of stability of the shoulders and hips.

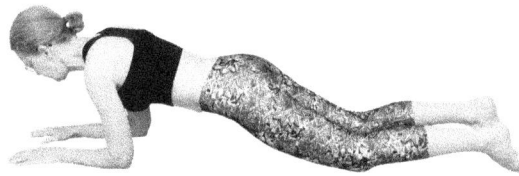
Figure 48

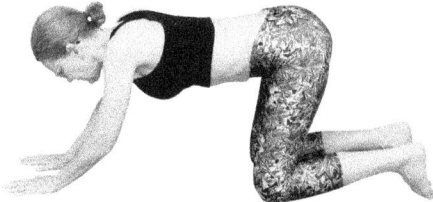
Figure 49

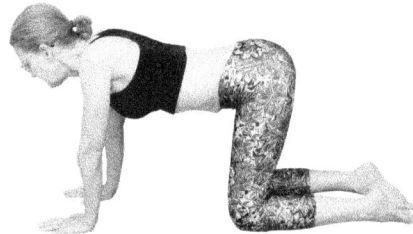
Figure 50

The second more mature strategy of transitioning from lying on stomach to quadruped requires more core, hip, and shoulder stability than the first strategy. Figure 51 shows weight shifting onto the right side of the body, which allows positioning of the left arm and leg in preparation for weight shifting and acceptance onto the left side (Figure 52). A full weight shift onto the left hand and leg frees up the right side to complete the transition into quadruped (Figure 50).

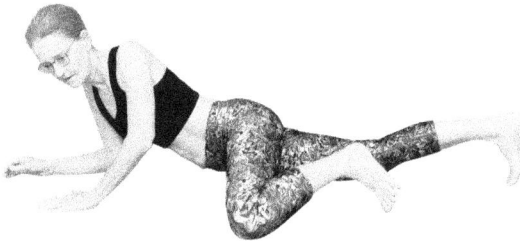
Figure 51

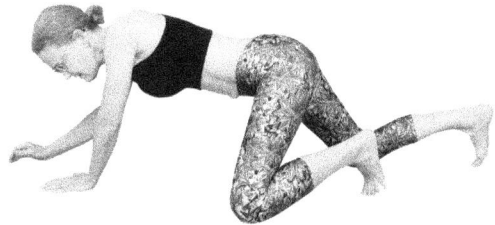
Figure 52

The quadruped position offers the opportunity to practice mobility of the lumbar spine and pelvis that may be used for weight shifting in sitting. Figures 53, 54, and 55 show three positions of the spine: neutral (slight extension or lordosis), extended (lordotic), and flexed, respectively.

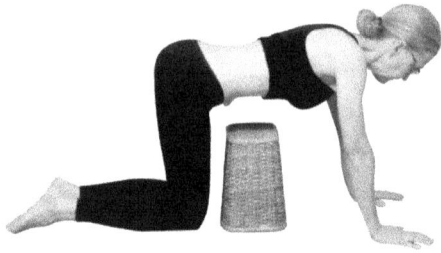

Figure 53

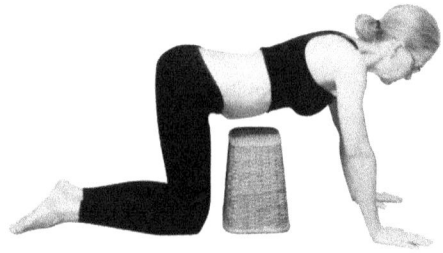

Figure 54

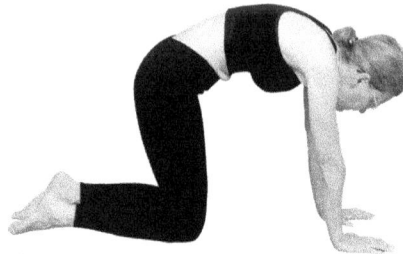

Figure 55

Core, hip, and shoulder stability are strengthened in quadruped by weight shifting from side to side, front to back, and combinations of these movements. Leg extension in quadruped may be part of core stabilization training to improve core and hip stability. Figure 56 shows good technique with the pelvis and trunk maintaining their neutral alignment. Poor core and right hip stability may cause either an excessive weight shift to the right (Figure 57) or poor weight acceptance of the right hip (Figure 58) demonstrated by the trunk and pelvis being rotated relative to the ground.

Eventually, the infant acquires enough core, pelvis, hip, and shoulder stability to perform mobility — crawling on hands and knees (Figure 59).

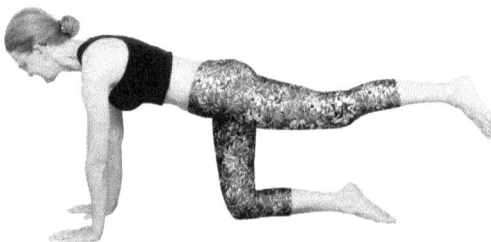

Figure 56

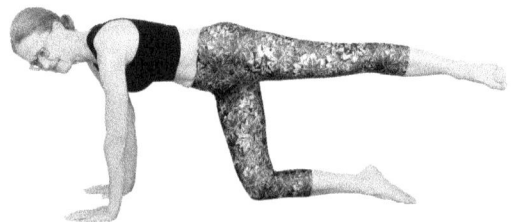

Figure 57

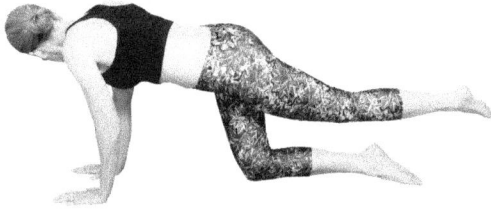

Figure 58

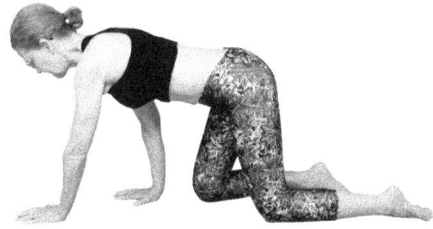

Figure 59

In the following sections we will analyze the movements that are part of everyday activities. Good performance of these basic postures and movement prepares the mover for good performance of skilled movements like dancing, kayaking, installing a new front door, or whatever movement goal they choose.

6 | Transitioning from sitting on the floor into quadruped

Getting from sitting on the floor into quadruped increases independence in infants and may help to maintain independence in adults. I have encountered many adults who were more afraid of not being able to get up from the floor than from falling. An infant who can transition from sitting into quadruped is rewarded with being able to explore their environment on their own terms (to the dismay of parents at times). For an adult, being able to transition from sitting on the floor into quadruped means having the option to crawl to a couch, chair, or bed to get up from the floor.

Because of the differences in the physical components of movement (flexibility, joint range of motion, strength, etc.) between an infant and an adult, there are some differences in the techniques each may use to transition from sitting to quadruped. Infants usually have more range of motion of the knees and hips, move quicker, and typically have less fear of losing balance than adults. Compare the steps involved in transitioning from sitting to quadruped in the infant (Figures 60, 62, 64, and 66) with the adult (Figures 61, 63, 65, and 67) described in detail below.

Position A (Figures 60 and 61): The infant (Figure 60) typically has greater right hip and knee flexibility than the adult, which provides more SSC of the right thigh and leg compared to the adult (Figure 61).

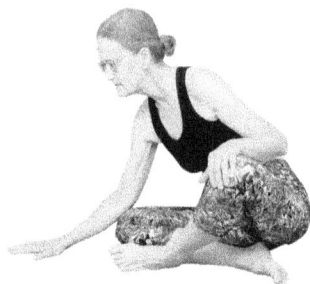

Figure 60

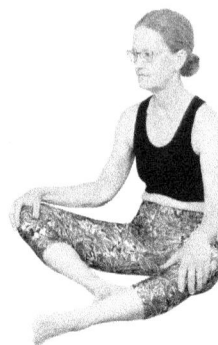

Figure 61

Position B (Figures 62 and 63): The infant (Figure 62) places their right hand forward and uses one hand for SSC and quickly starts to move the left hip. The adult (Figure 63) stabilizes themselves with two hands close to the body and slowly moves the left hip. With this added stability, an adult may be better able to stop the movement at any time. This may help to compensate for a slowing neurological system.

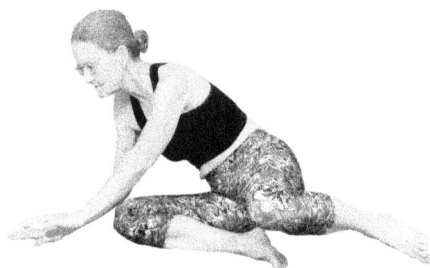

Figure 62

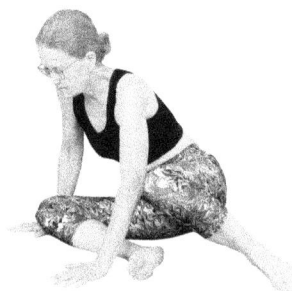

Figure 63

Position C (Figures 64 and 65): The infant (Figure 64) has their weight on the vertical right thigh and uses a large SSC of the right lower leg to push their COG up and forwards while quickly repositioning the left leg to prepare for the next part of the movement. The adult (Figure 65) uses the right hip muscles <u>and</u> their left foot to raise their COG to position the left leg. Since the adult has a higher COG than the infant, the adult is less stable than the infant. To compensate, adults may move slower and more deliberately using co-contraction of muscles around the right hip joint for stability.

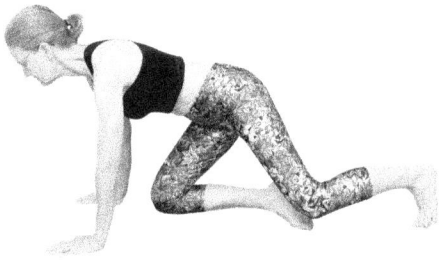

Figure 64

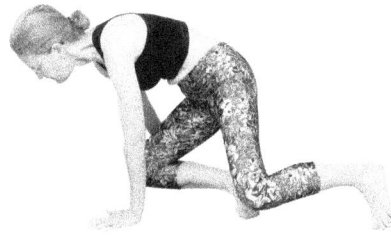

Figure 65

Position D (Figures 66 and 67): Because of the initial placement of the right hand, the infant (Figure 66) has a large BOS between the hands and the right knee. The infant's left foot is now positioned to propel the body forwards and crawling may begin immediately. In the adult (Figure 67), the pre-positioning of the hands close to the knees to gain stability in the early part of the movement resulted in a narrow BOS between the hands and the right knee – less stability. This may require the adult to perform several movements of their hands and knees to become stable before they use the left leg to start crawling forwards.

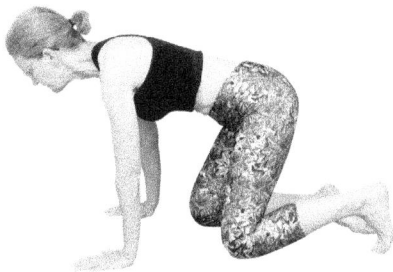

Figure 66

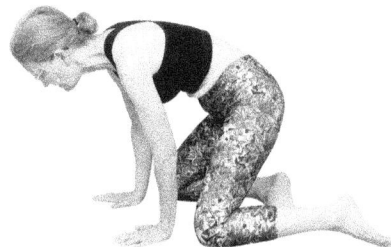

Figure 67

The above photos show that there is more than one strategy to reach the movement goal of getting from sitting into quadruped. The deficits in the SSC of the right thigh (Figure 61) may be improved by increasing right hip range of motion and muscle flexibility. Having better SSC may improve the quality of weight shifting. Repeatedly practicing a movement such as a weight shift without first improving what is causing the poor performance is like repeatedly making a cake with rotten eggs and expecting better results. *Good* practice makes *good* performance.

7 | Transitioning from quadruped to standing without furniture and using furniture

Transitioning from quadruped to standing may be done by transitioning through half-kneeling (Figures 68, 69, 70, and 71) and mini-squatting postures (Figures 72 and 73). Starting from quadruped (Figure 66), the left leg is brought forwards (Figure 68). Then the hands may be positioned on the left thigh to assist with straightening of the trunk (Figure 69). The positioning of the right toes prepares the body for the next phase of movement. In Figure 70, the toes of the back right foot are bent and are in position to provide a force to shift the body weight forwards and upwards. In Figure 71, the toes are straight or extended and are not as helpful to transition into standing. Pushing off the thighs (Figure 72) or off the chair (Figure 73) completes the transition to standing. The person in Figure 71 may decide to improve their thigh strength to improve their ability to transition from half-kneel to standing. However, if the deficits of the right toe are interfering with the movement, the person may benefit more by improving their right toe range of motion and strength.

Pearl of wisdom: the feet and toes in particular are important for weight shifting which is a fundamental for many movements like getting up from a chair, lunging, squatting, standing balance, and walking.

Figures 68, 69, 70, and 72 demonstrate the need for good SSC of the left foot for standing balance, the ability to generate a lot of force quickly, and timely coordination of weight shifting and weight acceptance of the legs. Using the chair (Figures 71 and 73) provides a larger BOS (distance between the hands and back of the heels versus the foot without the chair). Using the chair makes the movement more stable and less challenging in terms of balance and coordination.

View Figures 68-73 again and look for postural alignment, stability, SSC, COG within the BOS, weight shifting and weight acceptance by the hands and feet.

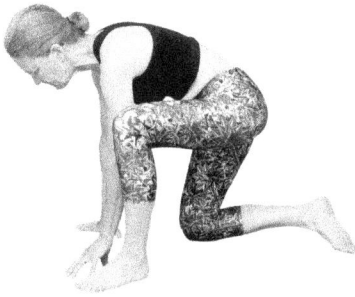
Figure 68

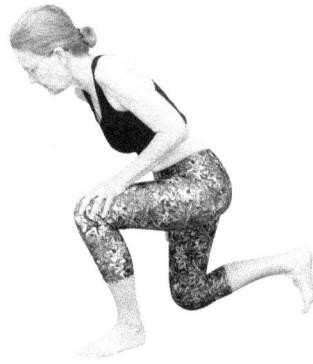
Figure 69

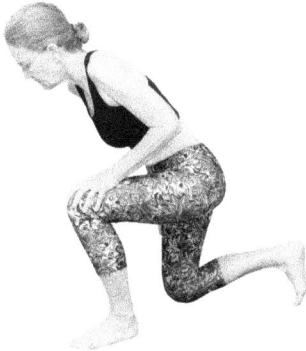
Figure 70

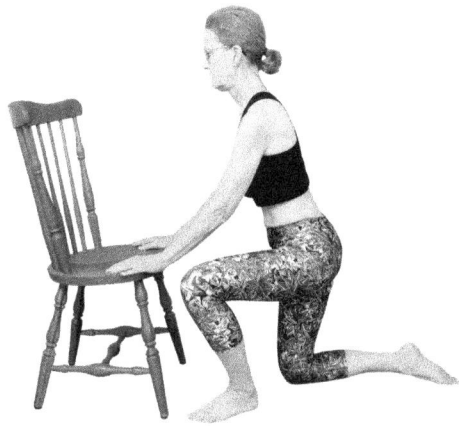
Figure 71

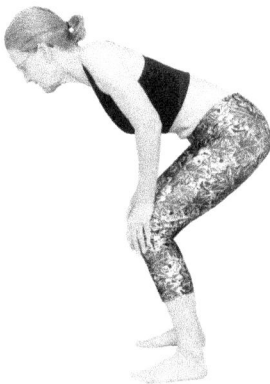
Figure 72

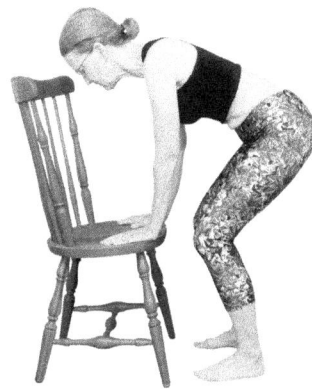
Figure 73

8 | Sitting in a chair — posture

We all know that we are supposed to have good posture when we sit. If you spend a large part of your day standing and walking, you may rationalize that a chair is for resting and you don't need to think too much about how you are sitting. On the other hand, if you spend most of your day sitting, you may not want to spend a lot of time having to think about how you are sitting. Unless you are completely supported when sitting and your hands are in your lap, you may benefit from learning some how-to's and how-not-to's of sitting.

Let's look at how-not-to sit, and then we'll move on to some ideas on how-to sit well. The postures in Figures 74, 75, and 76 show poor alignment of the head, neck, back, and pelvis. In Figure 74, the head is forward, and the low back is flexed which may lead to overuse of spinal muscles. In Figure 75, the head is forward and most of the bodyweight is on the low back which may cause excessive loading on low back disks. In Figure 76, the posture of the spine is better, and some bodyweight is supported by the upper thighs, but the feet have poor SSC. If you are in any of these positions (Figures 74, 75, and 76) for more than 10 minutes, you may feel that you are working too hard to hold up your arms, head, or back. In Figure 77, flexion at the hips shifts bodyweight forward and the arms can be supported on a work surface without needing to reach forward as in Figures 74 and 75. The good SSCs at the arms, upper thighs, and feet in Figure 77 allows for more even support of bodyweight with less reliance on spinal muscles to maintain good posture.

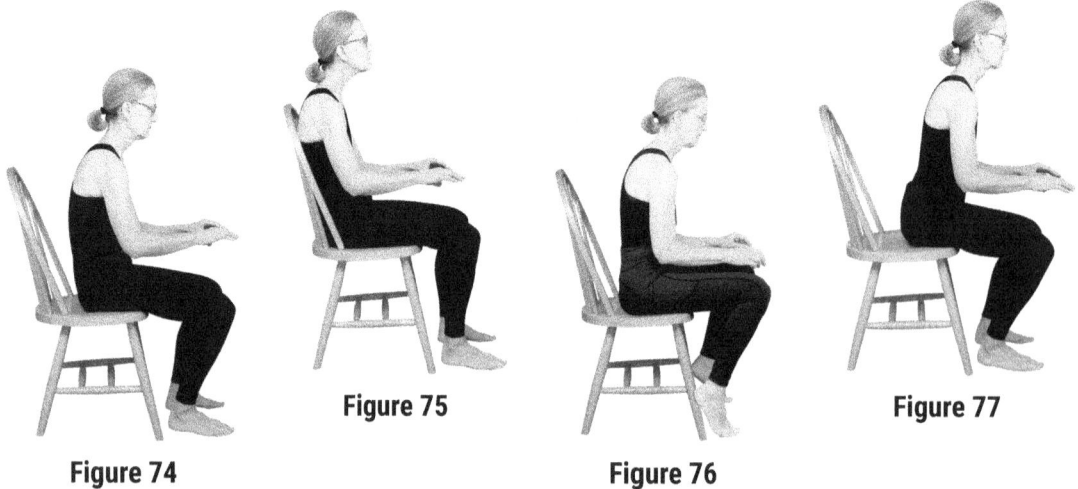

Figure 74

Figure 75

Figure 76

Figure 77

Perhaps the key to good sitting posture is more about weight shifting than staying in one position with perfect postural alignment. Staying in any one position, with good or poor alignment, may be a recipe for muscle fatigue. So, it may be useful to have the ability to change postures easily when sitting. Your 'genius car' knows that maintaining pressure on body parts for an extended time may reduce blood flow to tissue that provides life-sustaining oxygen. So, your survival instinct may say, "shift your weight frequently." The thought that "my leg is falling asleep," may be your brain telling you that a nerve or artery is being compressed and it would be a good idea to adjust your posture.

Some how-to's of sitting well might include (Figure 78):

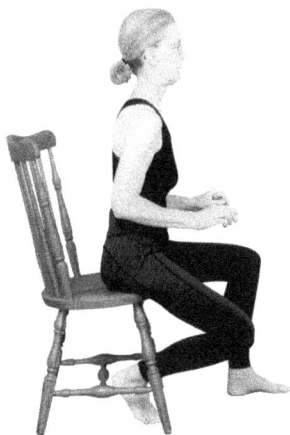 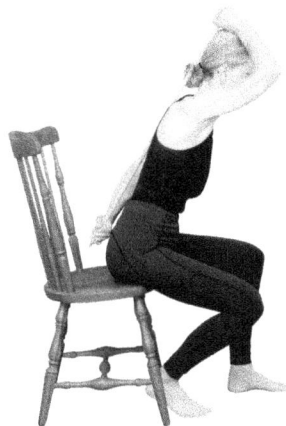

Figure 78   **Figure 79**

A. Distribute weight between the supported arms, the pelvis, and the legs and feet.

B. Maintain the spine in a neutral alignment (neck and low back slight lordosis or extension).

C. Take advantage of the size of the pelvic bones. (Figures 6 and 7 in Part 2). The pair of big bones behind the hip joint (ischial tuberosities) are large for bearing weight (sitting) which happens when you roll your pelvis forwards and sit up tall. If you slouch, you may be pressing on the little tail bones at the lowest part of the spine (coccyx).

D. Balance the head on the neck. When the head is forward (Figure 75), called forward head posture, the muscles at the back of the neck and head may be challenged to keep the head from falling forwards. Over time, a forward head posture may lead to a tension headache.

E. The arms as close to the trunk as possible and supported on a surface – COG of the arms within the BOS. Support as much of the forearm as possible, but at least the middle and lower parts of the forearm to help support the weight of the upper trunk.

F. One or both thighs angled downward to the floor to assist the spine to obtain a neutral posture (slightly lordotic or extended). As the thigh angles downwards, the lumbar spine becomes slightly lordotic. When the thigh is horizontal, the lumbar spine is in slight flexion and not in its neutral posture of slight lordosis.

G. Bend at the hips not the back when weight shifting and when transitioning to and from standing. This is called hip hinging (Figure 79).

H. Stagger the feet front to back to increase the BOS and position them as wide apart as the hips side to side. The back foot assists with forward weight shifting and the front foot assists with backward weight shifting. The left and right feet shift weight to the right and left, respectively.

I. Adjust chair height and position the pelvis near the front of the chair so one thigh angles downward. Modify the workstation to get close to the work and have arms supported. Adjust the height of the monitor so the head can be positioned in a neutral alignment, not flexed or extended.

9 | Moving to the front of a chair – weight shifting

There is more than one way to move forward in sitting to get out of a bed or up from a chair. A challenging way is to try to scooch both left and right buttocks forward together by pelvic thrusting or by pulling on a walker or piece of furniture that is in front of you. This requires the pelvis being stable and mobile at the same time. A more controlled and easier way to move forward in sitting might be to shift weight onto one buttock then move the opposite buttock forward (Figures 80, 81, and 82). Stability on one side allows mobility on the other, the same fundamental of movement that is used when reaching while lying on the stomach (Figure 43).

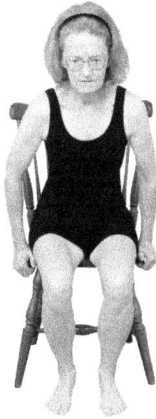 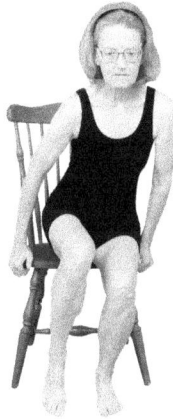 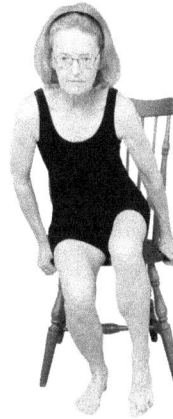

| Figure 80 | Figure 81 | Figure 82 |

10 | Transitioning from sitting in a chair to standing a) with hands, b) without hands

How many times a day do you perform sit to stand? You stand up from your bed, the toilet, your kitchen chair, to get out of your car, off a park bench, and up from the bottom step after you watched the sun set from your front porch. Not being able to get up from sitting to standing may be a barrier to independent living. Routinely performing sit to stand with good technique may help to maintain ankle, knee, and hip mobility and strength. On the other hand, transitioning from sitting to standing with poor technique may strengthen compensatory muscles and lock you into the compensation cycle. Movement memory is created for better or for worse. Lifting a laundry basket with poor technique by bending at the back rather than the knees may not be a good movement memory to rely on when picking up a runaway kitten. Storing good movement memory is probably a better strategy than having to undo a bad movement habit and then learn how to move a better way.

Have a look at the photos in Figures 83-90 before you read the following text to see if you can identify the movement fundamentals that are performed well and the ones that are performed poorly.

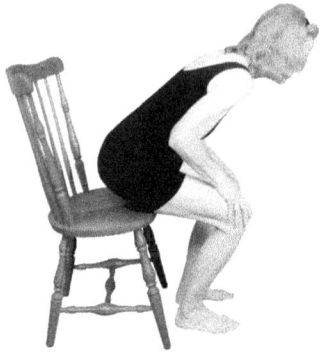

Figure 83

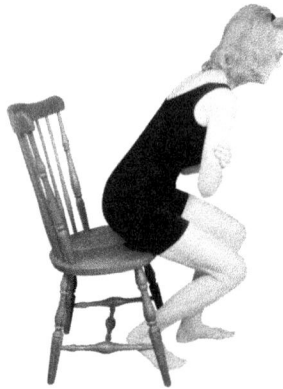

Figure 84

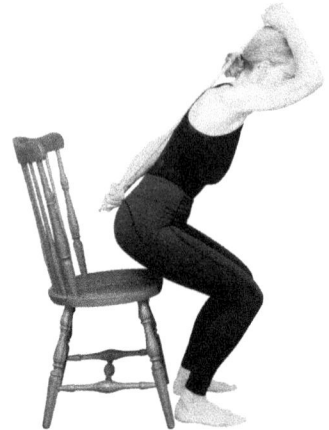

Figure 85

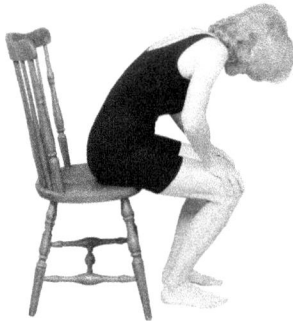

Figure 86

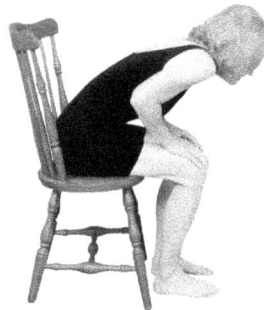

Figure 87

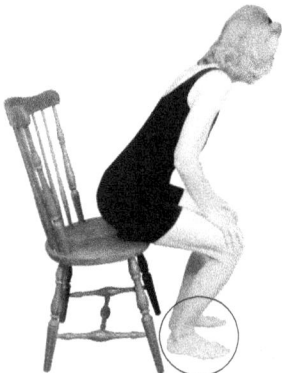

Figure 88

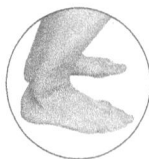

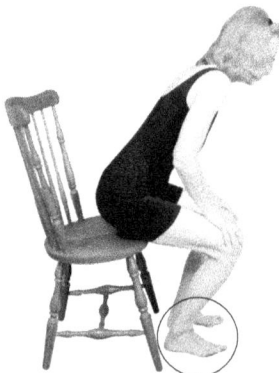

Figure 89

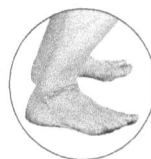

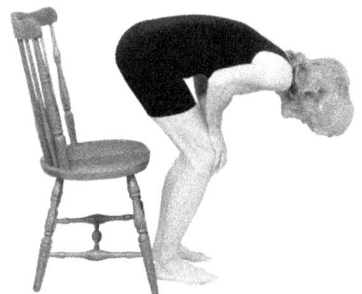

Figure 90

Figures 83-85 demonstrate good quality movement fundamentals. Figures 86-90 show deficits in movement fundamentals that may make the movement unsuccessful unless some body parts step up to compensate.

A. Start and end with good postural alignment. In Figure 86, poor spinal postural alignment may interfere with the COG moving forwards. Be prepared by training good stability – core and hip strength – and good mobility of the knees, ankles, and feet. If there is weakness in the calf, thigh, or hip muscles, the hands may be used to compensate by pushing off the support surface (Figure 83). However, using the hands to get up from sitting to standing makes them unavailable for functional tasks such as carrying and reaching.

B. Move forward in the chair so the COG can be positioned over the feet (not like Figure 87). Bend at the hips to move the COG of the trunk over the BOS of the feet (like figure 83, not like Figure 88). A staggered position of the feet, front to back (Figure 84), is good because it increases the BOS and provides the opportunity for the back foot to push the COG forwards. When the feet are staggered, the forward leg does most of the work raising and balancing the body, which requires good strength and balance. The foot alignment in Figure 84 may not be possible if there are limitations in the ankle range of motion of the back foot.

C. Maximize SSC of the feet. People that have neuropathy may have decreased or absent sensation of their toes, so their toes may not be in contact with the floor when performing sit to stand (Figure 89). This effectively makes the BOS front to back smaller making it more difficult to maintain balance (the COG within the BOS) as weight is shifted forwards. Using momentum to come into standing from sitting (Figure 90) may be unsafe when there are deficits in sensation of the toes because the toes may not be able to prevent the COG of the trunk from going too far forwards.

D. Use hip hinging to shift the weight of the COG of the body forward while maintaining good spinal postural alignment (Figure 85).

E. Rocking back and forth several times before getting up may help prepare body parts for weight acceptance and identify what may be interfering with a forward weight shift. Using momentum to get out of a chair may be a good strategy if it can be controlled. If a person's reaction times are too slow or there is weakness, using momentum to get out of a chair may not be safe.

F.   Look ahead rather than down (not like Figure 86) which may help to maintain spinal alignment and shift the COG forwards. In general, where the eyes go, the body follows as you may have been taught in a driver's education course.

G.   Ensure that the feet and legs are able and willing to accept weight. Thigh weakness and knee and foot pain may interfere with weight acceptance.

11 | Mini-squatting and hip hinging

The mini-squat is another activity that is done frequently throughout the day such as when taking a yogurt out of the refrigerator, getting water from the faucet while brushing your teeth, and reaching for an item that is on a bottom shelf. The muscles used for a mini-squat are the same ones that are used for sitting to standing. Hip hinging (Figures 79 and 85) compared to bending at the spine (Figure 86) relies on the larger leg muscles for control of the forward weight shift with a lesser demand on smaller spinal muscles. This is why bending at the hips rather than at the spine is recommended for safe lifting.

Mini-squatting is performed frequently in exercise programs because it is functional, and several muscle groups may be strengthened in one movement. Some people are taught to keep their weight on their heels when squatting and "don't let your knees go beyond the toes." But keeping the COG back on the heels is not what the body does naturally. Watch a toddler squat and see that their COG is over their midfoot and their knees are in front of their toes.

There are three reasons why having the weight on the midfoot – balanced between the toes and the heels – might be more appropriate than keeping the knees behind the toes with weight on the heels when performing squatting exercises: 1) Having weight on the toes provides the opportunity for safe and efficient weight shifting using the toes. Recall from Chapter 10 that a function of the toes is weight shifting. 2) When the COG is over the midfoot, there is usually less strain on the small back muscles and greater reliance on the large buttock and thigh muscles to control the squat, and 3) The body has a significant amount of movement memory of squatting and performing sitting to standing with weight on the midfoot starting from toddler days until the present time. Review these three points again and see how they exemplify the movement basics of safe, efficient, and pain-free and using movement memory to improve performance. The next time you get up from squatting or from a low seat (like the one in your bathroom for example), look and see if your knees are behind or in front of your toes. If your intent is to improve your function, it might be advantageous to exercise using postures that are like the ones that you use functionally throughout the day.

Observe the similarities in the photos of the position of the spine when rising from a chair with good technique by bending at the hips (Figure 91) and when mini-squatting using hip-hinging (Figure 92). The next two Figures 93 and 94 demonstrate poor spinal positioning for getting up from a chair and squatting. With poor technique (Figures 93 and 94), the spine is more vertical than in the previous figures (91 and 92) where hip hinging was used to perform sit to stand and squatting. In Figure 93, because the COG is too far back, the person may not be able to get up from the chair even with the use of the hands. In Figure 94, the person uses spine muscles to keep their COG on their heels and the spine is in a more vertical position like Figure 93. When squatting with the weight on the heels, there is increased demand on spinal extensor muscles. If you have back pain after squatting exercises, it may be that you are straining your back to keep your weight on your heels. This is not how your body typically moves when you get up from a chair or when you stand up from a squatting position after feeding your cat or dog.

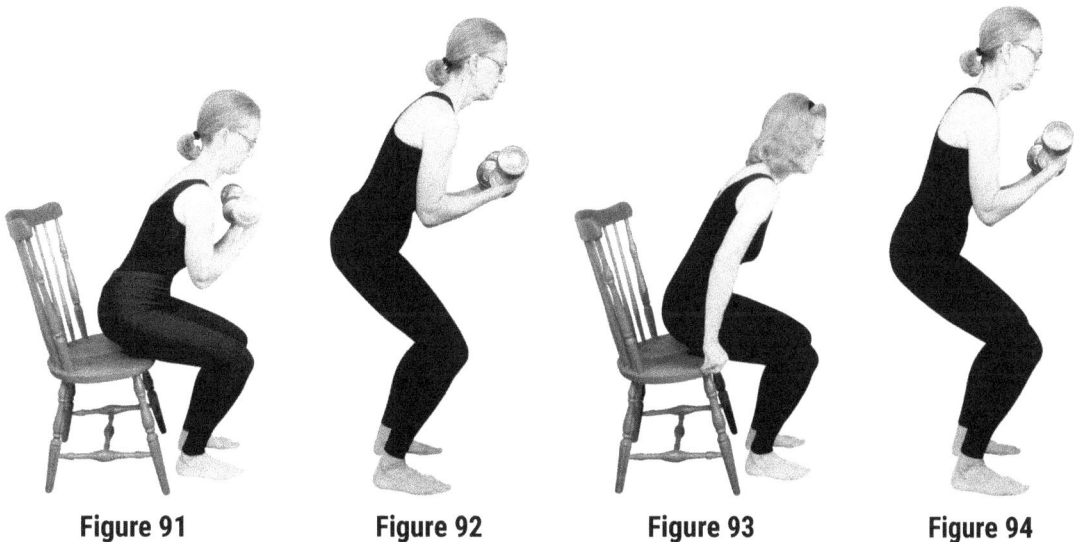

Figure 91   **Figure 92**   **Figure 93**   **Figure 94**

Good alignment of a mini-squat viewed from the front shows the knees joints in line with the ankle joints (Figure 95). This allows the knees to flex and extend easily, the way the knee joints were meant to function (Figures 9 and 10, Part 2). When the knee and ankle joints are in poor alignment (the knees closer together than the ankles as in Figure 96), knee stability is challenged. In this poor alignment, some of the thigh muscles may be needed to stabilize the knees, making them less efficient at performing their primary job of controlling knee flexion and extension.

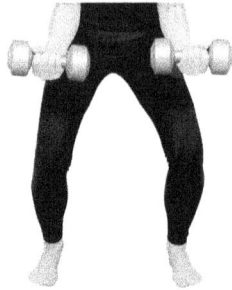 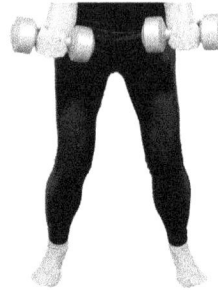

Figure 95   **Figure 96**

12 | Picking up shoes from the floor

The activity of picking up an object from the floor is like the mini-squat movement. Good postural alignment may be maintained by using hip hinging. Bending at the knees and hips, makes it is easier to keep the COG within the BOS of the feet so the arm can reach straight down to pick up the shoes (Figure 97). When using trunk flexion rather than hip hinging (Figure 98), the arm needs to reach forwards to pick up the shoes. In Figure 98, to keep the arm vertical to pick up the shoes, the trunk needs to shift forwards which may result in a loss of balance forwards. Like the previous activity (Mini-squatting and hip-hinging), bending at the back rather than the

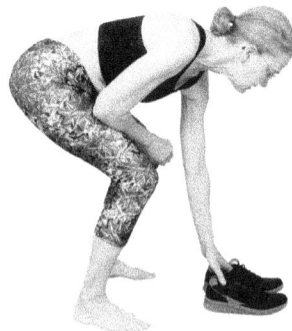 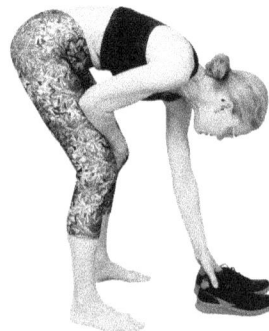

Figure 97   **Figure 98**

hips increases the demand on small back muscles (Figure 98) rather than relying on the larger hip muscles (Figure 97) to perform the movement. The right forearm on the thigh may assist raising the COG of the body to return to standing if both hands are not needed to lift the object.

13 | Standing on two legs

Compare the photos of good and bad standing posture. Good posture (Figure 99) shows the spine in a neutral alignment with the head resting on top of the neck and the weight of the body going through the midfoot. In the poor standing postures (Figures 100 and 101), several joints are positioned in end-range, which is undesirable because stability is gained by loading soft tissue rather than relying on the bony structure of joints. In Figure 100 the head is forward, the shoulders are rounded, the knees are hyperextended, and the weight of the body goes through the heels. In the 'sway back posture' (Figure 101), the abdomen protrudes forward, and the trunk leans or sways backwards. To balance the backward shift of the COG, the head moves forward, but the weight of the body still falls through the heels. In poor standing postures where

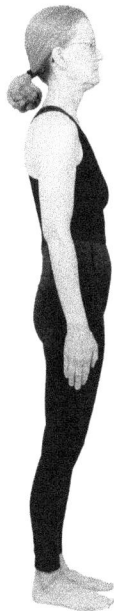 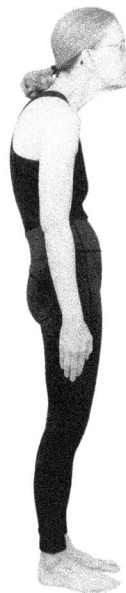 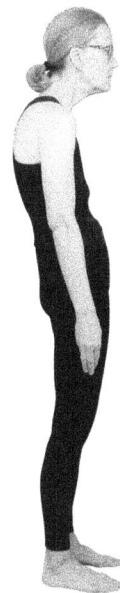

Figure 99 **Figure 100** **Figure 101**

the COG goes through the heels, weight shifting to start a movement may be more difficult. Contrast this poor standing posture to the 'ready position' that is used in sports like baseball or volleyball where the COG is on the forefoot so that the toes can perform weight shifting quickly to get to the ball.

14 | Standing on one leg – balance

Everyone has something to say about balance. "I have good balance." "I never had good balance." "I need to improve my balance." "I have better balance when I wear my sneakers." "Life is a balancing act." Yes, balance is an important skill to have. Every time you take a step there is a time when only one foot is on the support surface. This means that you need to be able to balance on one leg at least briefly when walking. If you can't stand on one leg for at least several seconds, then it might be safer to use a cane or a walker.

Balance Basics

Before we will look at photos and observe 'good' balance and 'not good' balance, let's apply the movement fundamentals to balance. Good balance when standing on one leg is achieved by:

A. Good **stability** of the hip to allow for good **mobility** of the feet for **weight shifting and weight acceptance**.

B. Good **SSC** the instant standing on one leg begins to be able to accept weight and keep the **COG within the BOS**.

C. The ability to maintain balance with good **postural alignment and endurance** for at least several seconds to allow time to recover from a loss of balance to help prevent a fall.

The movement fundamentals necessary for good balance that are highlighted above are based on the following:

A. the senses involved in controlling balance,

B. the three-legged stool concept of balance, and

C. ankle, hip, and stepping response strategies of balance.

Senses Involved in Balance

Vision, Vestibular, Proprioception, and Tactile

Vision tells your brain how your head is oriented relative to the horizon. When you lean your head or your whole body sideways (with your head still in line with your body), your vision tells your brain that your head is not vertical. If you were to close your eyes and lean your head or your whole body (with your head still in line with your body), your vision cannot give your brain any information about your head position. Fortunately, there are other sensors that can tell your brain about the alignment of your head and body – vestibular and proprioception.

The **vestibular** sensors in the inner ears tell your brain about head movements. The brain then signals muscles to activate to help you maintain balance. Some vestibular sensors detect horizontal and vertical accelerations of the head while others detect rotational accelerations. When turning your head to catch a baseball, the vestibular and visual systems work together to keep the ball in focus.

Proprioception is another sense that plays a role in balance. Proprioception refers to the sensations from muscles, tendons, ligaments, (soft tissue) and joints that provide information to the brain about where body parts are and how they are moving relative to each other. Proprioception may be referred to as body awareness. When you lean your head or your body sideways, your body senses stretch and other sensations from soft tissue and joints and updates your brain on body position and the relationship between body parts.

Tactile sensors in skin sense light touch, touch pressure, pain, temperature, and vibration. Tactile sensors tell your brain what parts of your foot are in contact with the support surface, the amount of pressure and/or pain on each part of the foot, and if your foot is slipping on the support surface. The tactile sense is responsible for providing information to the brain on support surface contact, the fourth movement fundamental. SSC is important because it impacts weight shifting and weight acceptance, the fifth and sixth movement fundamentals, and balance.

In Chapter 29, it was mentioned that to challenge a movement, close the eyes. When the eyes are closed, the visual information that the brain uses for balance is not available. This puts a higher reliance on the vestibular, proprioceptive, and tactile senses. If these sensors are not providing accurate and timely information to the brain, there may be a loss of balance when the eyes are closed.

The Three-Legged Stool Concept of Balance

Have you ever tried to level a four-legged table when the floor is uneven? A century or so ago, farmers milked cows while sitting on three-legged stools to make it easier to balance while sitting when a barn floor wasn't even. How successful will you be at keeping a bicycle standing up without using a kickstand – the third leg for balance? Using three legs, not two and not four, is the best strategy for balance especially when the ground is uneven.

How does the three-legged stool concept apply to balance? The three legs of your 'three-legged stool' are the big toe area, the little toe area, and the heel area. Increasing the BOS or the distance between the three points increases stability. Clowns can lean far forwards because they wear long clown shoes that keep their COG within their enlarged BOS. To lessen stability, decrease the BOS as anyone who has worn stiletto-heeled shoes can probably tell you. BOS also may be decreased when there is fear/pain-avoidance such as after spraining an ankle, stubbing the big toe, or trying to avoid a pebble in your shoe when you walk. As the BOS gets smaller, the COG has a greater likelihood of going outside the BOS which may result in a loss of balance. The moral of the story is: have as many parts of your foot available as possible to maximize your BOS to help with your balance.

The Ankle, Hip, and Stepping Response Strategies of Balance

There are three strategies of balance – ankle, hip, and stepping response – and they are used in three different situations.

In the ankle strategy of balance, the ankle wobbles to help maintain balance, but the hips, arms, trunk, and head stay relatively still. The ankle strategy is used when there is good SSC of the foot on a stable surface or there are small challenges to balance such as being slightly nudged.

In the hip strategy of balance, large movements of the hip are used to help maintain balance. The hip strategy is used when the foot has decreased contact with the support surface or there are significant challenges to balance like being moderately nudged. This may explain why there is excessive sway of the hips when people walk when wearing high-heeled shoes.

In the stepping strategy of balance, a person needs to take steps to regain balance. The stepping strategy is used to help prevent a fall when there is a major challenge to balance like tripping over a toy or pet, or responding to a very large nudge.

Standing on One Leg

To assess the ability to stand on one leg, the person ideally should be barefoot, eyes open, arms crossed in front of their body or relaxed at their sides, with the trunk and head in good alignment. The instructions are "bend your knee keeping your thigh in line with your body." Anything that deviates from that alignment suggests that they may be a compensation for a balance problem.

The good balance in Figure 102 shows good postural alignment from head to toe. The compensations for poor balance shown in Figure 103 may be a forward head posture, rounded shoulders, mild lumbar flexion, and bringing the non-stance thigh forwards. Balancing on one leg should be done by ankle muscles because the support surface is stable and the person is not being nudged (ankle strategy), but the person in Figure 103 is controlling their balance by using their head, trunk, and non-stance hip (hip strategy). Good balance viewed from the front (Figure 104), shows a trunk that remains vertical relative to the pelvis. Compensations for balance deficits viewed from the front show the trunk side bending towards the stance leg (Figure 105) or away from the stance leg and the arms coming away from the body (Figure 106).

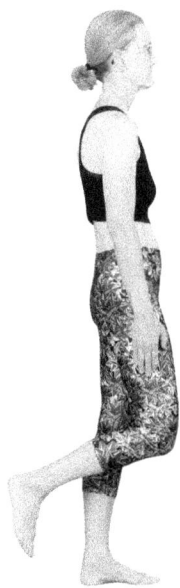

Figure 102

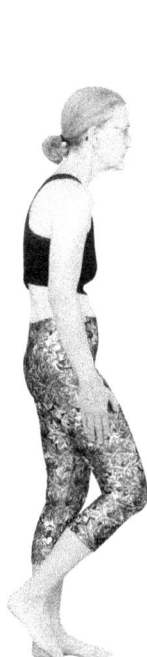

Figure 103

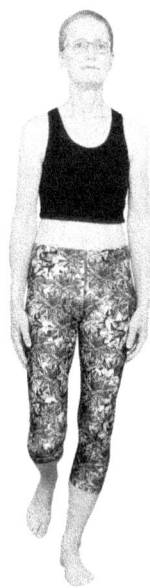

Figure 104

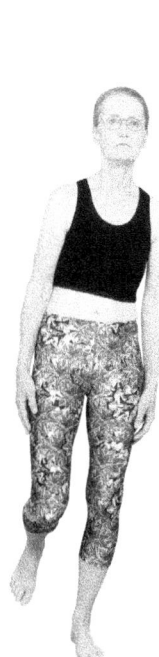

Figure 105

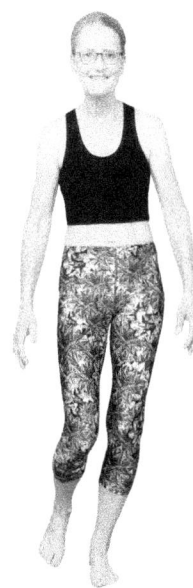

Figure 106

When observing balance, it is important to look at the contact between the foot and the floor the instant the non-standing foot comes off the floor. If any part of the standing foot comes off the floor even briefly, this suggest there may be a deficit in SSC which may impact balance.

Close-up photos of the foot and ankle show good (Figure 107) and not-so-good (Figures 108, 109, and 110) floor to foot contact at the first instant of standing on one leg. In the good balance of Figure 107, all the toes are in contact with the ground. In the not-so-good balance in Figures 108, 109, and 110 there is unloading of the big toe, toes 2,3,4,5, and the lateral ankle and 5th toe respectively at the first instant of standing on one leg.

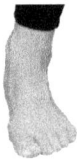 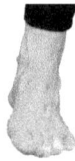 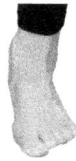 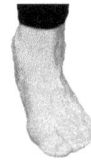

Figure 107   **Figure 108**   **Figure 109**   **Figure 110**

When the brain senses a deficit in SSC from pain, weakness, movement memory, etc., it may delay the weight shift and weight acceptance which may result in compensatory movements. Perhaps you have experienced pain in a toe or a leg while walking, and the very next step you did not have pain. Your brain very quickly created a new movement plan for you so you were able to walk without sensing pain. 'Genius!'

What Might Be Done to Improve Balance?

One possible answer has two parts: the 'what' and the 'why'. First identify *what* movement fundamental is not being performed well, and then hypothesize *why*.

Are there **postural alignment, stability, and endurance** deficits and if so, what is causing them?

Is there **stability** of the hips and **mobility** of the feet and ankles?

Is the **COG** outside the **BOS**, and if so, why?

Since **SSC** is important for balance, strategies that improve SSC such as decreasing or eliminating foot pain, or using footwear with better SSC may be beneficial.

Another way to improve balance might be to perform activities that challenge control of **weight shifting and weight acceptance**. The key word is control. Balance requires good coordination – good timing of muscles contracting and relaxing. Improving the ability to regain control of balance quickly by challenging balance at functional speeds addresses the weight shifting and weight acceptance fundamentals.

The following two functional activities of lunging and reaching benefit from having good floor to foot contact prior to achieve good weight shifting and weight acceptance. It helps to be able to walk well before you run, and also to stand well on one leg before you try lunging or reaching.

15 | Lunging forward – reaching

Lunging is performed by taking a step and shifting body weight onto the leading leg. Good lunging technique forward (Figure 111) is demonstrated by maintaining good postural alignment, shifting the COG within the BOS, good SSC of the forward foot, good weight shifting onto the forward leg by bending the forward knee, and good weight acceptance by the forward leg. Poor lunging technique (Figure 112) is demonstrated by excessive extension of the spine.

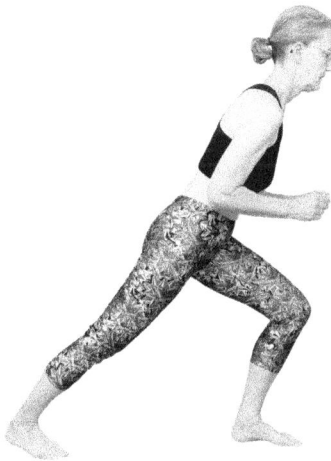

Figure 111

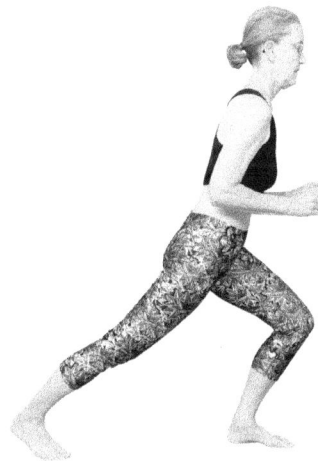

Figure 112

The activity of taking a jacket off a chair is an opportunity to practice good lunging technique to develop good movement memory (Figure 113). The poor technique in Figure 114 gives you a visual of how-not-to take a jacket off a chair.

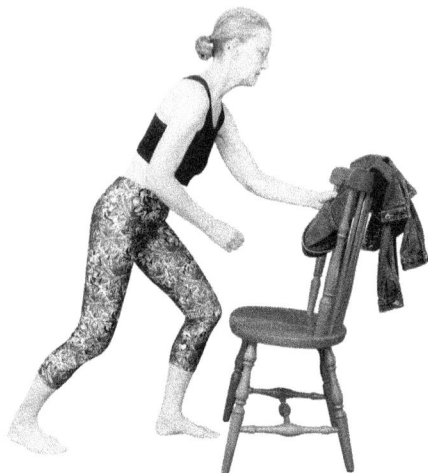 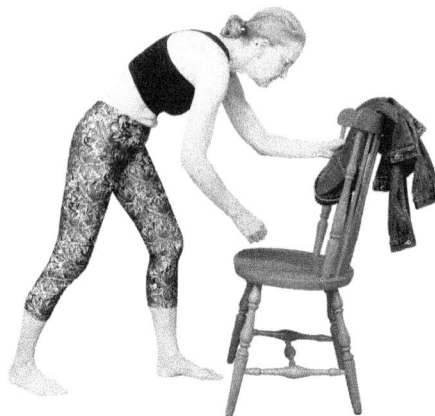

Figure 113   **Figure 114**

16 | Lunging to the side – reaching

Good performance of reaching to the side (Figure 115) is demonstrated by maintaining good postural alignment, increasing the BOS by turning the hips and taking a step to the side, good SSC, good weight shifting, and good weight acceptance of the leading right leg. Poor performance of lateral reaching (Figure 116) is demonstrated by the poor postural alignment, turning and bending of the upper trunk rather than the hips, a small BOS, decreased SSC of the leading leg with the weight shifted to the outside of the right foot, minimal weight shifting to the right side, and minimal weight acceptance onto the right leg. Compare the position of the right arms in the two figures. In the good technique shown in Figure 115, the right elbow is bent (flexed) and the person's COG has shifted closer to the towel. In the poor technique shown in Figure 116, the right elbow is straight (extended) and there is little weight shifting of the person's COG towards the towel. In addition, the spine is flexed and rotated in Figure 116 which may cause increased stress on shoulder and back muscles compared to Figure 115.

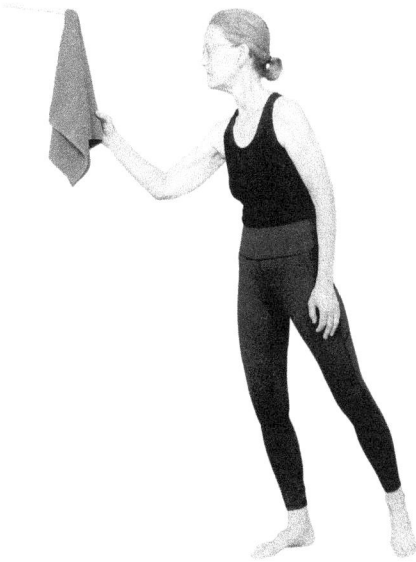

Figure 115

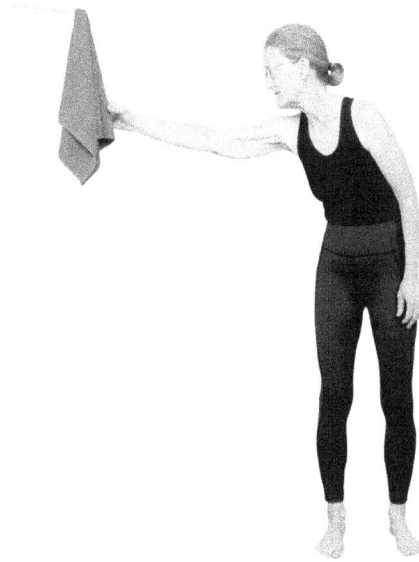

Figure 116

Having the ability to perform the above 16 activities well, provides a good foundation for higher level, skilled movements. 'Good practice makes good performance:' 1) good postural alignment, stability, and endurance, 2) good stability then good mobility, 3) maintaining balance by keeping the COG within the BOS, 4) good SSCs, 5) using good SSCs to shift body weight while maintaining good postural alignment, and 6) good weight acceptance while maintaining good postural alignment and balance.

On to Part 4 for some tips on how to be a better teacher of movement to yourself, your family, colleagues, patients, and clients.

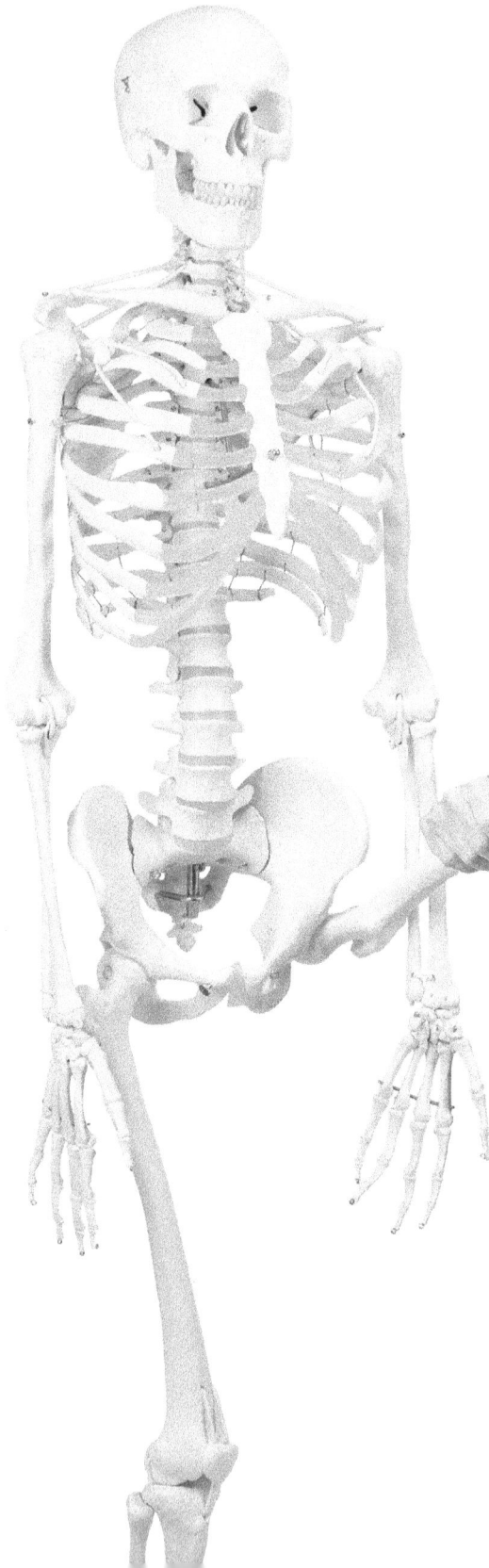

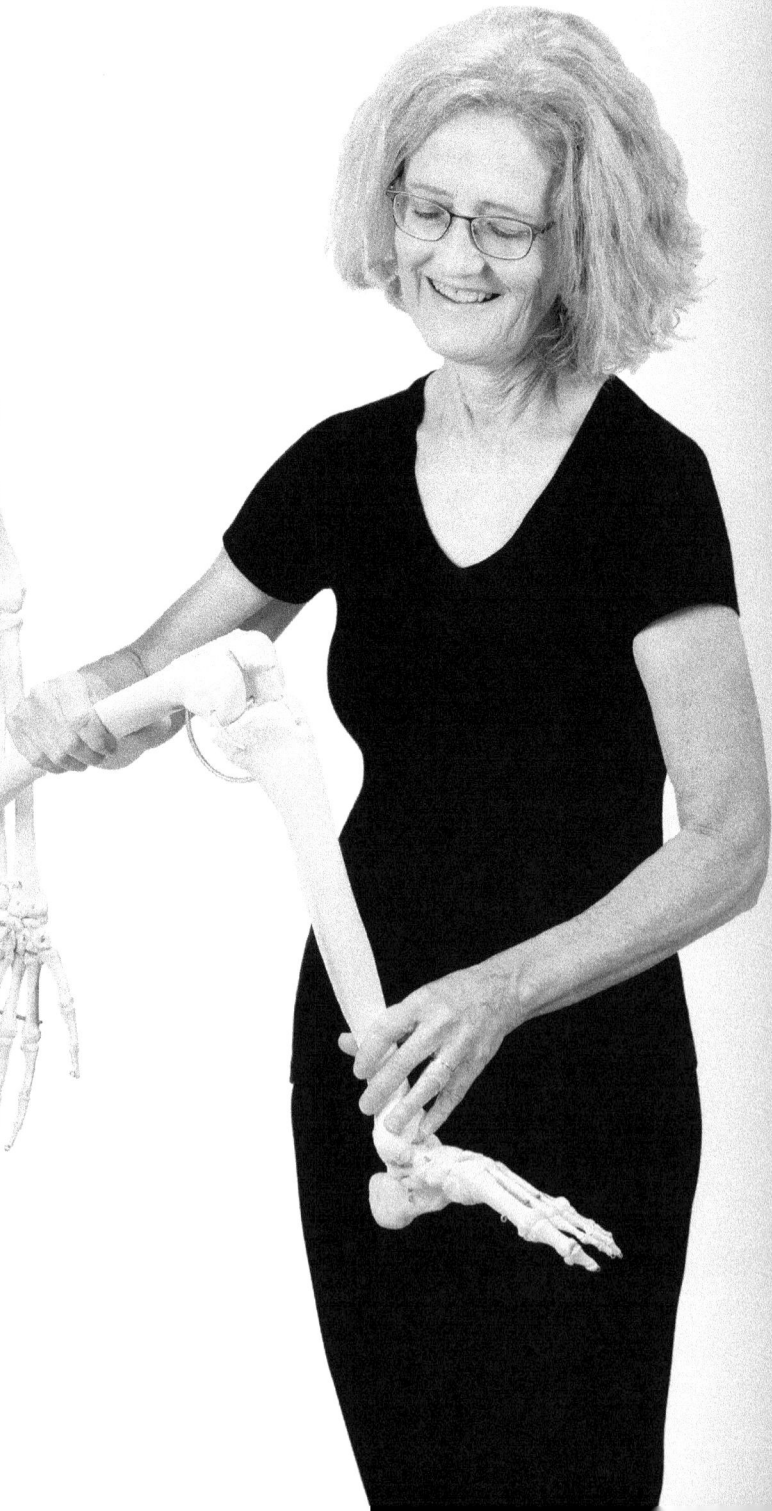

4

Teaching Movement

There are many opportunities for you to be a teacher of movement. You may be a healthcare provider, personal trainer, coach, physical education teacher, parent, home health aide, supervisor on an assembly line, furniture salesperson, a designer of car seats, or perhaps yourself when you are learning how to bowl or perform a new dance.

The learner may be your family member, your colleague, a member of the cheerleading squad, an apprentice carpenter, your patient, your client, or yourself.

When I first started teaching, I knew that knowing a lot was important, but I was lacking a good process for how to deliver knowledge. Many people know how to move well. However, because you know something well, does not necessarily mean you know how to teach what you know well. As you read through this chapter, I hope you will begin to appreciate that teaching involves many components just like movement.

These are the topics of teaching movement that will be presented in Part 4:

1. Learning Movement
2. The attributes of an effective teacher
3. Strategies for Solving Movement Problems
4. The process of change and habit formation
5. How not-to's of teaching movement
6. How-to's of teaching movement

CHAPTER 31

Learning Movement

Bloom's Taxonomy of Learning was first introduced in 1956[35] and since then has been expanded and revised.[36-38] Bloom's taxonomy is a system of learning that starts from basic abilities and progresses through stages building on the competencies achieved at lower levels. Bloom's taxonomy has three areas or domains of learning: cognitive, psychomotor (technical), and affective. Thinking. Doing. Feeling.

In Part 2 Knowing, you had the opportunity to learn or *know* about movement in the cognitive domain. Part 3 Doing provided information on the psychomotor domain of movement. The third, affective domain of learning about movement, was presented in Part 1 in terms of motivation, rewards, and valuing movement. The goal of Part 4, Teaching Movement, is to help you to be a better teacher of movement in all three domains. Effective teaching begins with the learner being introduced to knowledge at a basic level like definitions of terms, then progressing to higher levels of understanding, then application of the knowledge with competency being demonstrated at each level. Recall my chemistry class example of the need to be competent at the basics before being able to apply them to solve a problem.

Two things to keep in mind when teaching movement are a) to not skip any levels and b) make sure there is competency at one level before moving on to the next one. If you have a learner who is confused, frustrated, not motivated, or not learning, it may be because a level of learning was skipped or the learner did not demonstrate competence before advancing to the next level.

The following paragraphs show how movement can be taught in the cognitive, psychomotor, and affective domains of learning.

Cognitive Domain (*Knowing*)

In Part 2, body parts and their functions were listed and concepts like compensation, fear/pain-avoidance, and fatigue were explained. The analogy of a car compared to the human body was used to teach concepts of preventative maintenance of the body. Chapter 25 presented information on fundamentals of movement and how movement develops.

Psychomotor Domain (*Doing*)

Chapter 30 used photographs to show postures and movements to learn about identifying good and poor techniques. A progression of learning in the psychomotor domain would be to have someone perform a posture or movement and receive guidance as necessary.

Affective Domain (*Feeling*)

The affective domain concerns inter- and intra-personal intelligence, communicate skills, and readiness to learn and change.

Chapter 5 discussed making a choice to learn more about the movement system and barriers to changing movement habits. A progression in the affective domain would be to take responsibility for changing postures and movements to help decrease pain and/or improve performance.

Summary

Teachers have the potential to be role models in all three learning domains: cognitive, psychomotor, and affective. You may have heard the expression 'monkey see, monkey do'. Children especially are sensitive to non-verbal communication and may mimic parental behaviors even before they learn how to talk. Demonstrating good postures is a good way to reinforce verbal messages.

In addition to a thorough knowledge of the topic, an effective teacher explains why the learner needs to know the information that is being presented. By encouraging questions and discussions on the why's and how's of moving better, patients and clients can gain experience in the process of solving movement problems. Thus, besides learning what to do to move better, the learner becomes familiar with a process of how to address future movement concerns.

An effective teacher takes the time to assess the level of the learner in the cognitive, psychomotor, and affective domains and addresses the learner's expectations. Fortunately, learners of movement are usually well-motivated because of their movement limitations and the desire for a good outcome.

Challenges to learning in the affective domain might be demonstrated by someone who doesn't accept guidance well, or who ignores compensatory movements or overloading of body parts. To improve the learning experience when a patient or client appears frustrated, the teacher can initiate a conversation to help identify the cause(s). Perhaps the teacher did not detect a deficit in the learner's movement components, or the learner was not provided with appropriate guidance on how to perform movements correctly. Maybe there was a communication barrier between teacher and learner. Or, perhaps the teacher's directions or explanations were not understood by the learner and a different approach is needed to convey the information.

In sum, teaching movement engages cognitive, psychomotor, and affective domains of learning and benefits from ongoing assessment and modification to best meet the learner's goals.

CHAPTER 32

Attributes of an Effective Teacher

The process of teaching is based on respect, trust, acceptance, memory, willpower, and kindness.[39] If you think about the teachers in your life that were most memorable, they probably had some or all these attributes. The learning experience may be more positive if the learner has these attributes as well. In that regard, the teacher might benefit from knowing and be able to describe their learner.

What is the **physical** condition of the learner? What are their medical and movement histories? What are their resources in terms of time, energy, and finances?

What is the **emotional** maturity of the learner? How well do they self-assess? What is their learning style? Do they prefer to observe a movement many times, then perform it, or would they prefer to try a movement immediately after seeing it and refine it with repetition? Are the learner's beliefs about how they want their body to function realistic? Are they aware of their physical, emotional, cognitive, and spiritual strengths and weaknesses? What is their sensitivity to touch – do they avoid or accept guidance via touch? Are they a risk-taker or are they more cautious? Do they have any fears that may interfere with learning movement?

What is the learner's **cognitive** level of functioning? How able are they to receive and understand information using words or word pictures? Are they able to follow and recall directions?

Spiritually, has the learner given serious thought to their goals and are the goals reachable based on their physical, emotional, and cognitive abilities? How well does the learner accept constructive criticism?

A teacher of movement:

A. has an appreciation for the physical, emotional, cognitive, and spiritual attributes of the learner,

B. is knowledgeable about the process of learning and changing,

C. is effective in communicating the process and path for successful learning,

D. can share and demonstrate knowledge,

E. can assess competency of the learner, and

F. can help the learner to stay engaged in the learning process.

CHAPTER 33

Strategies for Solving Movement Problems

Besides Bloom's taxonomy, there are two other strategies that are sometimes used for solving movement problems: the shotgun (try everything at once) approach, and the trial-and-error (randomly try potential solutions) approach. The following example compares the shot gun and trial-and-error approaches with the strategy of using Bloom's taxonomy to solve a movement problem.

Tennis player asks: Why do I have pain in my shoulder when I serve a tennis ball?

Tennis player thinks: Maybe my racquet is too heavy, I am not throwing the ball high enough, or I am weak or not flexible enough.

She uses the shot-gun approach and borrows a lighter racquet, goes to the gym, lifts weights, and stretches her arm, and throws the baller higher, but still has the same pain.

Tennis player thinks: Maybe I need new shoes.

She used the trial-and-error approach and buys new shoes, but she still has the same pain.

Let's see how the tennis player could use the affective, psychomotor, and cognitive domains of learning to help solve her movement problem. She could seek guidance (affective) to have her physical components and fundamentals of movement assessed (psychomotor). Using knowledge about the movement system, possible causes of her pain could be identified (cognitive) and appropriate interventions could be implemented to address the possible causes.

In sum, competency at fundamentals of movement – postural alignment, stability, and endurance, stability then mobility, center of gravity within the base of support, good support surface contact, weight shifting, and weight acceptance – is necessary before attempting highly-skilled activities where precision and speed are important for success.

CHAPTER 34

The Process of Change and Habit Formation

The purpose of this book is to share knowledge about movement so that people may be able to improve their ability to move safely and efficiently without pain. Applying the knowledge from this book to meet movement goals may require changing movement habits or creating new movement habits. Part of the process of moving better is to do enough repetitions so that movement becomes automatic, that is, it becomes a habit and part of movement memory.

What are your current movement habits? Do you stretch before activities, even work activities? Do you bend down to move something out of your way, or do you use your foot to push it? You may benefit from stopping bad movement habits and/or starting good movement habits.

Creating a movement habit involves the process of change which was presented in Chapter 6. When making a change, it is helpful to have a reminder of when to perform the new behavior. For example, if your goal is to run a 10K or hike with your social group, seeing your sneakers or your exercise equipment can be a reminder to engage in your exercise or movement program. Or, whenever you need to reach for something that is lower than your knee, you are reminded to bend your knees and use good postural alignment so you can meet your goal of safe, efficient, pain-free movement.

A barrier to creating a new habit might be that you haven't found the right incentive to change your behavior. The process of change also includes receiving frequent rewards. Rewards may be verbal such as being complimented by a teammate after completing a strenuous training session. Or, rewards may be more tangible such as treating yourself to a concert or sporting event after you reach your goal of winning a game or meeting your weightlifting goal.

Habit Formation and Movement Fundamentals

Table 6 lists some tips that may be helpful to make fundamentals of movement habitual and part of movement memory.

The goal is safe, efficient, and pain-free movement. *Know*, *do*, then make the doing a habit.

Table 6: Movement Habits

Fundamental of Movement	Habit
1. Good postural alignment, stability, and endurance	Make stretching a daily routine; learn and maintain good posture for all activities
2. Good stability then mobility	Use abdominal muscles to maintain good postural stability during transitional movements throughout the day
3. Maintaining balance by keeping your center of gravity within your base of support	Set up the environment so there is space for an adequate base of support; when reaching and moving, keep the center of gravity safely within the base of support
4. Good support surface contacts	Use appropriate non-slip footwear; be aware of potentially unsafe surfaces
5. Using support surface contacts to shift body weight while maintaining good postural alignment	Become aware of compensations due to pain or other issues; seek professional guidance to identify and address the causes of the compensations
6. Weight acceptance while maintaining good postural alignment and balance	Use fundamentals 1-5 in all movements to improve postural stability and endurance; create good movement memories

Some How-*Not*-To's of Teaching Movement

For a more pleasant experience for the learner:

1. Don't skip steps.

2. Don't overly complicate.

3. To prevent feelings of inadequacy, refrain from demonstrating movements that may be beyond the abilities of the learner.

4. Don't assume anything.

Some How-To's of Teaching Movement

To help improve engagement of the learner:

1. Tell the learner what you are going to do, do it, then tell them what you did.

2. Include enough content that is necessary and sufficient, but not too much to be confusing.

3. Use the body's sensory systems to communicate information: visual cues, words, word stories/analogies, or touch (if appropriate).

4. Ask open-ended versus yes/no questions which tend to provide more accurate information about the concerns of the patient or client.

5. Repeat and review until the learner provides feedback of understanding either verbally or by demonstration.

6. Encourage questions and open communication.

7. Encourage self-assessment.

8. Update goals when necessary.

9. Use intellectual honesty: if you don't know something, say so and try to find the knowledge.

10. Be humble and be kind.

11. Respect the 'genius car'.

12. Have FUN!

In Conclusion

This book began with T.S. Eliot's quote, *"We shall not cease from exploration and the end of our exploring will be to arrive where we started and know the place for the first time."*[1] I hope you had a pleasant journey exploring 'What **YOU** Need to Know to Move Better' and that your exploration has brought you to a more complete understanding of your movement system.

Wishing you the all the joys and benefits of movement. Take care of and enjoy your 'genius car.'

*Scan the QR code or visit **https://bit.ly/KCYourBodyinMotion** to access larger, printable versions of Appendices A through D.*

APPENDIX A
Trauma, Surgery, Skeletal Asymmetries

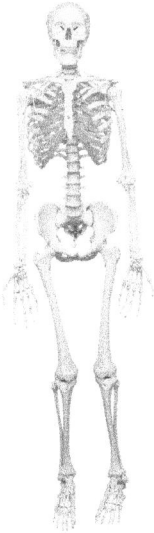

Trauma *Fall, struck by an object, sports/work injury, car accident, fracture, sprain, bruise, abrasion, etc.* (label each corresponding number on the skeleton)

	Injury	Body Part	Age
1.			
2.			
3.			
4.			
5.			
6.			
7.			

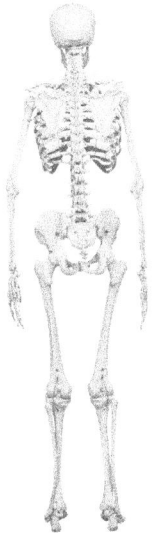

Surgery (label each corresponding letter on the skeleton)

	Body Part/Surgery	Age
A.		
B.		
C.		
D.		

Skeletal Asymmetries *Scoliosis, leg length inequality, etc. (*label the corresponding * on the skeleton)*

* _____

Pain, Weakness, and Other Symptoms

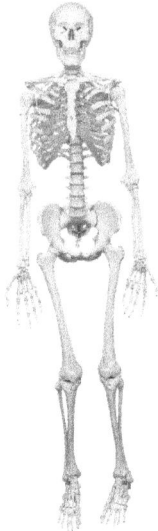

Pain (label each corresponding number on the skeleton)

Body Part	Age
1.	
2.	
3.	
4.	
5.	
6.	
7.	

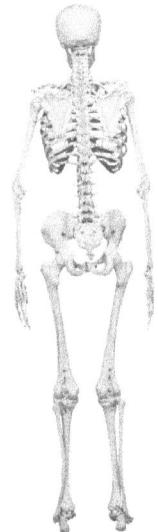

Weakness (label each corresponding letter on the skeleton)

Body Part	Age
A.	
B.	
C.	
D.	
E.	
F.	
G.	

Other Symptoms *Numbness, dizziness, vertigo, etc.*

1. _____
2. _____
3. _____

Place an 'X" to the left of the number on the list if the symptom has resolved.

Interventions to Improve Movement

Body Part/Movement Problem	Intervention/Provider/Dates

1. _____
   Outcome (circle one):   Better   Worse   No change

2. _____
   Outcome (circle one):   Better   Worse   No change

3. _____
   Outcome (circle one):   Better   Worse   No change

4. _____
   Outcome (circle one):   Better   Worse   No change

5. _____
   Outcome (circle one):   Better   Worse   No change

6. _____
   Outcome (circle one):   Better   Worse   No change

7. _____
   Outcome (circle one):   Better   Worse   No change

Use of Braces, Casts, Splints, Orthotics, Assistive Devices, etc.

Device/Body Part	Dates of Use

1. _____
2. _____
3. _____
4. _____

Lifetime Activity Level

Fill in the bubble to indicate your activity level

Activities

AGE	ACTIVITY	MINIMAL		MODERATE		VERY
0–9	Home	○	○	○	○	○
	Recreation	○	○	○	○	○
10–19	Home	○	○	○	○	○
	Work	○	○	○	○	○
	Recreation	○	○	○	○	○
20's	Home	○	○	○	○	○
	Work	○	○	○	○	○
	Recreation	○	○	○	○	○
30's	Home	○	○	○	○	○
	Work	○	○	○	○	○
	Recreation	○	○	○	○	○
40's	Home	○	○	○	○	○
	Work	○	○	○	○	○
	Recreation	○	○	○	○	○
50's	Home	○	○	○	○	○
	Work	○	○	○	○	○
	Recreation	○	○	○	○	○
60's	Home	○	○	○	○	○
	Work	○	○	○	○	○
	Recreation	○	○	○	○	○
70's	Home	○	○	○	○	○
	Work	○	○	○	○	○
	Recreation	○	○	○	○	○
80's	Home	○	○	○	○	○
	Recreation	○	○	○	○	○
90's	Home	○	○	○	○	○
	Recreation	○	○	○	○	○

NOTES

NOTES

NOTES

Acknowledgments

I am very grateful to

- All my patients who have shared their movement concerns with me. Thank you for your perseverance in wanting to know how your body works and for asking questions to help you make wise movement decisions. Your thoughtful remarks that you wanted other people to benefit from what you were learning *before* they got injured motivated me to write this book.
- Teachers and colleagues who generously shared their knowledge, experience, and expertise on the movement system, physical therapy, and how to be an effective educator.
- Janine Logan, editor and healthcare writer for her editing skills and enthusiasm.
- Kim Poulos Lieberz and her talented team at KGI Design Group (Michelle Fink, Lindsey Hund, and Nora Ryder) for their creativity and expertise at presenting information visually.
- Stephanie Larkin at Red Penguin Books for getting this book into your hands.
- My family and friends for their encouraging words throughout the writing process.

Special thanks to my husband Joseph for his photography expertise and continuous support throughout the 'what YOU need to know to move better' journey.

References

1. Eliot, T. S. (1943). Little Gidding in *Four Quartets*. New York, Harcourt, Brace, and Co.

2. Harburg, E. Y. (words) & Arlen, H. (music). (1939). *Follow the Yellow Brick Road*. From the movie *The Wizard of Oz*. Metro-Goldwyn-Mayer. Based on the book by Baum, L. F. (1900). *The Wonderful Wizard of Oz*. GM Hill Co.

3. Baum, L. F. (1900). *The Wonderful Wizard of Oz*. GM Hill Co.

4. Loane, M. (1911). *The Common Growth*. Kessinger Publishing, LLC. (Source is controversial.)

5. Franklin, B. (1735, February 4). Pennsylvania Gazette.

6. McGonigal, K. (2019). *The Joy of Movement*. Avery. An imprint of Penguin Random House LLC.

7. DeSchryver, A. M., Keulemans, Y. C., Peters, H. P., Akkermans, L. M., Smout, A. J., DeVries, W. R., & Berge-Henegouwen, G. P. (2005). Effects of regular physical activity on defecation pattern in middle-aged patients complaining of chronic constipation. *Scan J Gastroenterol* 40(4), 422-9.

8. Dainese, R., Serra, J., Azpiroz, R., & Malagelada, J. R. (2004). Effects of physical activity on intestinal gas transit and evacuation in healthy subjects. *Am J Med 116*(8), 536-9.

9. Willeumier, K. (2020). *Biohack Your Brain*. (Chapter 4). William Morrow, an imprint of HarperCollins Publishers.

10. Breuning, L. G. (2016). *Habits of a Happy Brain*. Adams Media.

11. Burnett, D. (2018). *Happy Brain. Where Happiness Comes From, and Why*. W.W. Norton & Company.

12. Moffat, M. & Lewis, C. B. (2006). *Age-Defying Fitness*. Peachtree.

13. Nelson, D. (2013). *The Mystery of Pain*. Singing Dragon.

14. Kubler-Ross, E. (1970). *On Death and Dying*. Collier Books/Macmillan Publishing Co.

15. Roosevelt, F. D. (1938). Inaugural Address March 4, 1933, in S. Rosenman (Ed.), *The Public Papers of Franklin D. Roosevelt, Volume Two: The Year of Crisis, 1933* (pp. 11-16). New York: Random House.

16. Bacon, F. (1597). *Meditationes Sacre*. Excusum Impensis Humfredi Hooper.

17. Levangie, P. K., & Norkin, C. C. (2001). *Joint Structure and Function*. (3rd ed.). F. A. Davis Company.

18. Morgan, D. (1988). Concepts in functional training and postural stabilization for the low-back-injured. *Topics in Acute Care Trauma Rehab 2*(4), 8-17.

19. Saint-Exupéry, A. (1971). *The Little Prince*. (p. 87). Harcourt Brace Jovanovich

20. Butler, D. S., & Moseley, G. L. (2013). *Explain Pain*. (2nd ed.). Noigroup Publications.

21. Richardson, C., Hodges, P., & Hides, H. (2004). *Therapeutic Exercise for Lumbopelvic Stabilization*. (2nd ed.). Churchill Livingstone.

22. Travell, J. G., & Simons, D. G. (1983). *Myofascial Pain and Dysfunction. The Trigger Point Manual*. (Chapter 2). Williams & Wilkins.

23. Bishop, M. D., Torres-Cueco, R., Gay, C. W., Lluch-Girbes, E., Beneciuk, J. M., & Bialosky J. E. (2015). What effect can manual therapy have on a patient's pain experience? *Pain Manag 5*(6), 455-64.

24. Xue, X., Ma, T., Li, Q., Song, Y., & Hua, Y. (2021) Chronic ankle instability is associated with proprioception deficits: A systematic review and meta-analysis. *J Sport Health Sci 10*(2), 182-91.

25. Bullock-Saxton, J. (1995). Sensory changes associated with severe ankle sprain. *Scand J Rehabil Med 27*(3), 161-7.

26. Rogers, R., & Hammerstein, O. (1951). From the song "Getting to Know You" from the musical play *The King and I*. Based on the book by M. Landon. *Anna and the King of Siam* (1944). Garden City Publishing Company.

27. Center for Disease Control and Prevention, STEADI – Older Adult Fall Prevention. https://www.cdc.gov/steadi/index.html.

28. National Institute on Aging, Falls and Fractures in Older Adults: Causes and Prevention. https://www.nia.nih.gov/health/topics/falls-and-falls-prevention.

29. Guerrasio, J. (2022). *Embrace Aging*. Rowman & Littlefield.

30. Linden, D. J. (2015). *Touch. The Science of Hand, Heart, and Mind*. (pp. 71-73). Viking. The Penguin Group.

31. Kenney, W. L., & Chiu, P. (2001). Influence of age on thirst and fluid intake. *Med Sci Sports Exer 33*(9), 1524-32.

32. Niebuhr, R. (1932). The Serenity Prayer. (Source is controversial). https://www.aa.org/sites/default/files/literature/assets/smf-129_en.pdf.

33. Davies, R. (1951). *Tempest-Tost*. (p. 127). Clark, Irwin.

34. Tscharnuter, I. (1993). A new therapy approach to movement organization. *Physical & Occupational Therapy in Pediatrics 13*(2), 19-40.

35. Bloom, B. S. (1956). *Taxonomy of educational objectives, Handbook I: The cognitive domain*. David McKay Co. Inc.

36. Krathwohl, D. R., Bloom, B. S., & Masia, B. B. (1964). *Taxonomy of educational objectives: The classification of educational goals, Handbook II: Affective domain*. David Mckay Co. Inc.

37. Simpson, E. (1972), *The Classification of educational objectives in the psychomotor domain: The psychomotor domain*. Vol. 3. Washington, D.C. Gryphon House.

38. Anderson, L. W., Krathwohl, D. R., Airasian, P. W., Cruikshank, K. A., Mayer, R. E., Pintrich, P. R., Raths, J., & Wittrock, M. C. (2001). *A Taxonomy for learning, teaching, and assessing: A revision of Bloom's taxonomy of educational objectives*. Pearson, Allyn & Bacon.

39. Highet, G. (1989). *The Art of Teaching*. Vintage Books. A Division of Random House.

Index

www.ingramcontent.com/pod-product-compliance
Lightning Source LLC
Chambersburg PA
CBHW051318020426
42333CB00031B/3397